Postpartum Depression and the Communicative Construction of Maternal Identity

Postpartum Depression and the Communicative Construction of Maternal Identity

Motherhood in Tension

Kelly M. Weikle

BLOOMSBURY ACADEMIC
NEW YORK • LONDON • OXFORD • NEW DELHI • SYDNEY

BLOOMSBURY ACADEMIC
Bloomsbury Publishing Inc, 1359 Broadway, New York, NY 10018, USA
Bloomsbury Publishing Plc, 50 Bedford Square, London, WC1B 3DP, UK
Bloomsbury Publishing Ireland, 29 Earlsfort Terrace, Dublin 2, D02 AY28, Ireland

First published in the United States of America 2026

A catalog record for this book is available from the Library of Congress

ISBN: HB: 978-1-6669-6112-6
ePDF: 979-8-216-26960-1
eBook: 978-1-9787-6745-4

Typeset by Integra Software Services Pvt. Ltd.

For product safety related questions contact productsafety@bloomsbury.com.

To find out more about our authors and books visit www.bloomsbury.com
and sign up for our newsletters.

To Ainsley and Landon.
It's never too late to pursue your dreams.

Contents

Acknowledgments

First and foremost, I want to thank my dissertation advisor Angela Hosek. Your mentorship has meant the world to me. I can still remember the first time I met you, at orientation for the doctoral program. My conversation with you is what made me sure I could go back to school as a mom, and you have continued to support me with your wisdom and guidance all the years since. I am in awe of your expertise, knowledge, and life advice. Thank you for leading me in the execution of this research and helping me turn my dissertation manuscript into the best it could be.

Thank you to my committee, Drs. Laura Black, China Billotte Verhoff, and Risa Whitson. Your expert guidance, direction, and support pushed me beyond my comfort zone and helped me become a better scholar. Thank you for your engaging feedback and questions throughout the dissertation process. Each of you brought something special to this project that ultimately made it what it is today. I cannot thank you enough for your commitment to me and my dissertation.

Thank you to those persons who helped me get the word out about my study. Becca, Michelle, Stephanie, and Ariel, thank you for your interest in my work and sharing my study with potential participants. Thank you to all those who shared my study information on social media and within their social circles.

Thank you to the women who participated in this study, who were willing to share their stories with me—stories that often left them in tears as they recollected times of struggle. So many times, you thanked me for doing this research. It is you who should be thanked. Without your willingness to share your personal stories, none of this would be possible. You are paving the way for a brighter future for those who struggle with PPD.

Thank you to all those people who were stuck listening to me talk about my research at networking events, children's soccer games, school events, and other get-togethers. Yes, you were involved in the knowledge-making process. Many times, as I spoke my thoughts out loud, I would make connections or see something in a new light based on responses from others. I truly value those conversations and the benefit they had on this research.

And finally, to Chris. Thank you for always encouraging me to follow my dreams and for your unwavering support. You are my rock.

Introduction

In the Disney film *Encanto*, the song "Surface Pressure" explores the emotional toll of familial role expectations, pressures, and constraints. Songwriter and composer Lin-Manuel Miranda shared that the "song inside the song" reflects how he was feeling during the uncertainty of the Covid-19 pandemic as he grappled with keeping his family safe, saying, "Who am I if I cannot be this role that everyone sees me as?" (Aswad, 2022, np). This inward question became the line: "Who am I if I don't have what it takes?"

That question—*Who am I if I don't have what it takes?*—is what I asked myself after I had my son, my second child, in June 2017. I don't know precisely when my postpartum depression set in, but what I remember most about the fall of 2017 is that I don't remember anything at all. It was like I was going through the motions and living life with those glasses that simulate driving while intoxicated. Things felt really foggy. I was home full-time, caring for a three-year-old and a newborn. I had some wonderful friends who were also home with their small children, but I still felt so alone. Nap time was my reprieve, but my newborn wouldn't nap unless I was holding him, and my three-year-old was on a nap strike. I was always tired. I constantly felt like I didn't have what it took to be a mom of two.

Miranda's lyric articulates something many of us quietly wrestle with: the fear that we might not be able to live up to the roles we've taken on in life. That's part of why "Surface Pressure" struck such a chord, especially with those stepping into new family roles. The most intense feeling I had when I had postpartum depression was feeling like I was a bad mom and a bad partner. As I slowly spoke to other women about their experiences with postpartum depression, I learned that I wasn't alone in feeling like a failure. These conversations led to my interest in the connection between societal idealization and expectations of motherhood and experiences of postpartum depression.

In this book, I'm focusing on motherhood and the identity shifts that accompany postpartum depression. I don't think it's presumptuous to say that, at some point, most mothers have asked themselves a version of Miranda's question. Society expects mothers to have no cracks, no breaks, make no mistakes, and never buckle under pressure. But what happens when we *do* feel like we're buckling, when we can't meet the demands society puts on us, or when we cannot even recognize ourselves? How do our interactions with others, our behaviors, and our ideas about mothering impact our identity as we go through postpartum depression? These are the questions I began to ask and eventually decided to pursue in my research.

A Brief Background on Postpartum Depression in the United States

The period after birth is a time of immense change for mothers. The term "matrescence" is gaining traction as a way to describe the developmental and transitional period that women experience following childbirth (Athan, 2024). During this time, a woman undergoes changes in various domains of life, including physical, neurological, social, and cultural, among others (Athan, 2024). As women give birth, even beyond their first birth, they face fundamental identity challenges as well as physical challenges. Women must navigate the complex web of their changing identities within their families, friendships, roles, work, physical appearance, and health.

Furthermore, women face many health risks as they grow, give birth, and care for their children. The most common health complication for women following the birth of their child is postpartum depression (Rafferty et al., 2019). Postpartum depression occurs in the period after the birth of a child and up to twelve months post-birth. Despite the common occurrence of postpartum depression, it remains a condition that is not fully understood, fraught with stigma, and goes highly undiagnosed and untreated (Rafferty et al., 2019). Additionally, postpartum depression has adverse effects on the mothers who experience it (Slomian et al., 2019). Women experiencing postpartum depression live in a world of shame, guilt, rage, despair, and other negative feelings that can have lasting psychosocial consequences (Beck, 2006).

Postpartum depression is the most known perinatal mood and anxiety disorder (PMAD), but there is a range of PMADs that can affect women during pregnancy and following the birth of their child. The types of PMADs that can occur during pregnancy include depression, anxiety, obsessive-compulsive disorder (OCD), and bipolar disorder (Postpartum Support International [PSI], 2024). After childbirth, mothers can experience post-traumatic stress disorder related to traumatic birth experiences, postpartum depression or anxiety, OCD, or bipolar disorder. Additionally, postpartum psychosis is a rare condition where mothers experience hallucinations, confusion, mania, and thoughts of harm toward themselves or others. Postpartum psychosis occurs in 0.1–0.2 percent of births and manifests suddenly, usually within the first two weeks following the birth (PSI, 2024). Unlike postpartum psychosis, postpartum depression is not a rare condition; rather, it is a common health complication faced by mothers following the birth of a child.

There is no definitive statistic describing rates of postpartum depression in the United States compared to other countries because of cultural differences regarding conceptualizations of depression and practices of after-birth care for mothers. Worldwide reported rates of postpartum depression vary from 0.5 percent to 60 percent globally (Abdollahi et al., 2011), although extensive transcultural research has indicated that postpartum depression is a universal experience (Beck et al., 2006). The rate of women affected by postpartum depression in the United States also varies by report, depending on scales and qualifications used to study the experience. Research by the Centers for Disease Control (2021) found that 1 in 8 women experience symptoms of postpartum depression nationally. Still, this rate varies by state and can be as high as 1 in 5 women (Bauman et al., 2020). Other researchers have found elevated postpartum depressive symptoms in 8–39 percent of women in the United States (Beck et al., 2011).

Alarmingly, in a national study, Beck and colleagues (2011) found that 63 percent of mothers screened positive for depressive symptoms at around seven months after giving birth, and 42 percent screened positive for depressive symptoms six months after that. McMahon and colleagues (2008) found that more than half the women diagnosed with postpartum depression in their study continued to experience episodes of depression beyond twelve months postpartum. Furthermore, healthcare experts estimate that half of women who experience postpartum depression go undiagnosed and untreated (Rafferty et al., 2019). Based on the research, postpartum depression is prevalent, underdiagnosed, and can last beyond the postpartum period.

While the cause of postpartum depression is not fully understood (Mollard, 2014), medical professionals believe the condition results from a combination of physical and emotional factors (National Institute of Mental Health, 2024). Indeed, risk factors are a mix of biological and psychosocial conditions. In the United States, predictors for postpartum depression include "low social support, a history of depression, life stress, prenatal depression, low education, and race/ethnicity" (Beck et al., 2011, p. 428). Other risk factors include familial history of depression, an unintended or unwanted pregnancy, domestic or family violence, being on Medicaid insurance or uninsured, low economic status, smoking and substance abuse, single status, being under thirty years of age, or having previous children (Rafferty et al., 2019). Furthermore, geographic status also presents as a risk factor; in the United States, women in rural versus urban settings are at a 21 percent higher risk of experiencing perinatal depression, accounting for race, ethnicity, and maternal age (Nidey et al., 2020).

Following the delivery of the child, additional risk factors manifest, including experiencing stressful life events during pregnancy or the early postpartum period, a traumatic birth experience, preterm birth or the infant being admitted to neonatal intensive care, and breastfeeding problems (Rafferty et al., 2019). Beck and colleagues (2011) found two prominent predictors of postpartum depression: elevated post-traumatic stress symptoms and low levels of health-promoting behaviors. Researchers have also linked attachment theory to postpartum depression, finding that the severity of depression symptoms at four months postpartum and an "insecure state of mind regarding attachment" in the mother independently predicted depression beyond twelve months postpartum (McMahon et al., 2008, p. 201). Women who gave birth during the Covid-19 pandemic were at increased risk for developing anxiety during pregnancy or in the postpartum period (Hessami et al., 2020). The risk factors associated with postpartum depression are numerous and wide-ranging. The outcomes of postpartum depression also vary.

In their meta-analysis of studies examining maternal and infant outcomes of untreated maternal postpartum depression, Slomian et al. (2019) identified several notable adverse outcomes associated with postpartum depression. First, research has shown that mothers with postpartum depression report more negative mood and psychological outcomes in the long term than those without postpartum depression, including lower self-esteem, lower mood scores, and feeling less happy and angrier (Slomian et al., 2019). Women who experience postpartum depression are more likely to have anxiety disorder and depression one year after childbirth than those who do not experience postpartum depression. Women with postpartum depression feel a lower quality of life, more stress, and less household functioning (Slomian et al., 2019). Higher levels of postpartum depression in mothers are associated with an increased prevalence of suicidal ideation and thoughts of self-harm.

Concerning effects on the child, maternal postpartum depression predicted more overall physical health concerns for infants and more childhood illnesses (Slomian et al., 2019). Additionally, postpartum depression can hurt maternal-infant interaction during the first twelve months of the infant's life (Beck et al., 2006). Consequently, left undiagnosed, postpartum depression can have long-term adverse effects on mother, child, and the mother-child relationship (Beck, 2006).

Previous research investigating subjective experiences of postpartum depression makes it clear that women face identity challenges such as identity loss and maternal failure in their postpartum depression experience (e.g., Beck, 1993; Mollard, 2014; Scharp & Thomas, 2017; Vik & Hafting, 2012). While we know postpartum depression does manifest in identity challenges for mothers, the way a communicative perspective conceptualizes identity offers the ability to comprehend more fully why and how these challenges manifest. Examining postpartum depression through a communicative identity framework can help researchers and professionals understand this condition and how it affects mothers, identify problems mothers face as they navigate their family roles, and identify best practices for supporting mothers during challenging times.

Contributions

The high rate of postpartum depression in mothers, the variety of risk factors, and the effects of untreated postpartum depression on both mother and child render a need to move beyond focusing on causes/risk factors of postpartum depression to explore how to best support mothers in managing challenges they may face within their postpartum depression, including challenges in their identities. In response to this need, the claims I make in this book are grounded in my analysis of interview data and shaped by my interpretation of these findings in conversation with existing research. Through the book, I argue that:

- Identity gaps are present as women experience postpartum depression. The mothers I spoke with navigated tensions between their experiences, their expectations, the expectations of others, their relationships with romantic partners, family members, and friends, directives from healthcare providers, and the dominant ideologies of what constitutes good motherhood.
- In the Communication Theory of Identity (CTI), the relational layer can be separated into two layers: ascribed relational identity and relational identity. Separating these two concepts can help researchers explore the complex nature of how messages from others and interpersonal relationships impact identities.
- The communal layer of identity goes beyond the individual and impacts relationships. Scholars may consider the communal identity as interpenetrating the relational layers. Within my interviews, I identified the communal identity of "mother" present in recalled conversations between spouses and between mothers with their own mothers.

- Looking at postpartum depression through an identity perspective offers a unique and meaningful way to advance understanding of the condition.

Additionally, in the last chapter, I propose empirically grounded practical support solutions for mothers facing mental health struggles in the postpartum period.

This book is about women's experiences during one of the most challenging and potentially traumatic periods of their lives. The claims presented above, and the data and analysis presented throughout this book, come from my dissertation, completed in 2022, where I explored women's identity experiences and tensions in the context of postpartum depression. I approached the experience of postpartum depression from a communicative identity standpoint. I framed my analysis through the CTI (Hecht et al., 2005) to explore and discuss identity frames and gaps in women who experienced postpartum depression. I conducted this research through an interpretive framework, where I used phronetic iterative analysis (Tracy, 2020) in interviewing sixteen women who had experienced postpartum depression (readers can find a more detailed description of my methods in the appendix of this text).

I use phrases such as "women" and "mothers" throughout the book when discussing the women I interviewed; however, it is essential to note that I use these terms in reference to the specific women I spoke with rather than making broad, generalizable claims about *all* women or *all* mothers. The experiences reconstructed here are valuable and important, representing one picture of women's experiences but not the whole picture. Indeed, the goal of interpretive research is to present a story that helps us better understand a phenomenon, not to explain all of a phenomenon (Tracy, 2020). My goal is to achieve resonance with readers and to make a significant contribution to the understanding of identity, motherhood, and postpartum depression (see Tracy, 2020 for criteria for high-quality qualitative research). Next, I provide a brief overview of the theoretical lens that framed my research and interpretations.

Theoretical Perspective: The Communication Theory of Identity

To better understand identity challenges through the lens of a communication framework, I used the CTI as a sensitizing framework for my research and analysis. The CTI situates communication and identity as two sides of the same coin, where "identity is formed, maintained, and modified in a communicative process and, thus, reflects communication" (Hecht et al., 2005, p. 31). Indeed, in CTI, communication and identity are not separate constructs. CTI centers the role of communication in identity formation and enactment, claiming identity is formed, maintained, and modified through communication, and externalized through communication (Hecht et al., 2005).

While other theories, such as Social Identity Theory (Tajfel, 1974), have looked at the influence of identity on communication, CTI takes it a step further by saying communication is internalized as identity. There are two ways this happens. First, drawing on symbolic interactionism, CTI says that symbolic meanings of phenomena are created and exchanged through social interaction. Identity forms when relevant symbolic meanings are internalized or attached to an individual (Hecht et al., 2005). Second, people place themselves and/or are placed into categories, and through social interaction, they validate whether those categories are relevant to them (Hecht et al., 2005). This cyclical process is what links communication and identity. CTI draws upon several influences, including classical conceptualizations of identity from various cultures, ideas from the Enlightenment and postmodernism, identity theory, and SIT (Hecht et al., 2005). Additionally, CTI was developed and applied in multiple paradigmatic traditions, including post-positive, interpretive, and postmodern (Soliz & Colaner, 2018).

Central to CTI is the idea that identity is discursive (Hecht et al., 2005). Therefore, identity is not something that exists only within the mind; rather, identity can be situated both within the individual and among people (Hecht et al., 2005). This layering of identity conceptualizations serves as an analytical device for the theory (Hecht, 2015). CTI articulates four layers where identity resides: the personal, the enacted, the relational, and the communal. In CTI, layers are dialectic; both changing and stable, subjective and ascribed (Hecht, 2015). While the layers of identity can be and are analyzed separately, they cannot function independently in reality (Hecht et al., 2005).

CTI uses the term "interpenetration" to articulate how the layers of identity interrelate (Hecht, 2015). Identity layers interpenetrate, but they may not always be in alignment. Discrepancy among the layers is referred to as an "identity gap" (Jung & Hecht, 2004). Indeed, Jung and Hecht argue that gaps are always present to some degree; what to consider is the degree and type of gap and the implications of the gaps for social relations and well-being. Identity gaps can emerge between two or more layers, such as a personal-enacted gap or a personal-relational gap (Jung & Hecht, 2004), or within one layer, such as a communal-communal gap (Bergquist et al., 2019).

CTI conceptualizes identity gaps as the result of communication and/or as variables influencing communication outcomes (Hecht et al., 2005). Jung and Hecht (2004) found high negative correlations between the personal-relational and personal-enacted identity gaps and the communication outcomes of communication satisfaction, feeling understood, and communication appropriateness and effectiveness. Additionally, identity gaps have been associated with negative psychological outcomes, such as depression (Jung & Hecht, 2008).

CTI has shown value in a wide range of contexts, including cultural identity, family identity, health identity, and sexual identity. Because identity gaps often occur when individuals adjust to new societal norms and expectations, CTI is a useful frame for studying identity formation and negotiation during times of change (Bergquist et al., 2019). Having a child is undoubtedly a time of change for mothers. CTI has also demonstrated its strength in helping scholars understand complex family forms (Soliz & Colaner, 2018). Additionally, CTI has been used to look at illness identity, and "CTI assumes that identity is formed through interaction, making it a viable theoretical framework for advancing development of illness identity research" (Hecht et al., 2005, p. 270).

As women become mothers, they must adjust to the day-to-day individualized experience of caring for an infant and the new societal norms and expectations associated with their new role. Furthermore, research has made clear that mothers experiencing postpartum depressive symptoms experience significant effects on their identity. Therefore, using CTI to understand how mothers navigate identity formation and negotiation while experiencing postpartum depression can offer insight into the relationship between identity, social interaction, and postpartum depression.

Previous research points to identity tensions and loss faced by mothers in the postpartum period. Since identity tensions have implications for psychological and relational health and well-being (Bergquist et al., 2019; Jung & Hecht, 2004, 2008), studying identity tensions within the postpartum depression experience could offer pathways to understanding how the condition manifests and how to support women as they go through postpartum depression. Furthermore, prioritizing the role of communication may be helpful in understanding how mothers communicatively manage their identity within the postpartum depression context.

Overview of the Book

As previously mentioned, I interviewed sixteen women who had experienced postpartum depression within the last ten years. I introduce them throughout the book (pseudonyms used) by sharing their quotes, stories, and experiences. I include more information about demographics in the appendix. In the first chapter, I focus on the experience of postpartum depression. To understand how identity manifests, I felt it was important first to understand what symptoms the women I spoke with faced as they experienced postpartum depression.

I spend the following four chapters describing how identity manifested through various layers for the women I interviewed: through their changing selves, their communication and behavior, their expectations of motherhood as influenced by cultural scripts, and, finally, through their relationships and the messages they received from others. In each chapter, I begin by highlighting the experiences of one of the women I interviewed or by sharing my own experience. I then describe the common threads of how identity manifested within the layers, including additional examples to support my claims. Next, I discuss identity gaps related to the layers in consideration. Finally, I conclude with some commentary on what the experiences and analysis presented reveal about the manifestations and tensions of identity in the postpartum experience, in conjunction with our existing knowledge from previous research.

In the last two chapters, I discuss the implications of my findings. First, in Chapter 6, I discuss how my study contributes to the understanding of identity as communicative and enhances our explication of the CTI. In Chapter 7, I discuss how to apply the findings to better support women and mothers, both in the healthcare field and within close relationships. In the Afterword, I share more about my own experience with postpartum depression and why I wanted to conduct this work. Finally, in the Appendix, I share a brief overview of my method and the limitations of the research.

1

Experiencing Postpartum Depression

Anxiety; have trouble making decisions; feeling empty, hopeless, overwhelmed; persistently doubting ability to be a good mother; frequent feelings of anger or rage; tired all the time; numb to feelings—feel like I'm looking at the world through cataract eyes; often angry at husband; never feel like a good mom at the end of the day; no resilience when things go wrong; just want to be alone; feel like I'm making life miserable for everyone around me/ruining [older child's] life; from [husband]: "defeatist attitude."

Right after [son] was born, I felt great, but by the time my six-week follow-up was coming up, I looked up symptoms of PPD, but I didn't have any, maybe like one, so I thought okay I'm good. I was going to mention something but then I got scared and didn't say anything. Summer was great, but I feel like I don't remember the fall or winter. Vacation, Christmas . . . Last Sunday I finally reached the point where I had to face the hard truth that I'm not myself. I feel silly for letting it go on this long but I also feel like I should be stronger than this. Scared to take medicine.

Two excerpts from a notebook I kept in 2017

I look back at what I wrote in that notebook and have to laugh (and cry). Of course I had postpartum depression! How did I not see it? How did no one else see it? Those notes about my postpartum depression were the last thing I wrote in that notebook. I almost threw the notebook away several times. I didn't want to be reminded of this experience that shook me to my core. In hindsight, I'm glad I saved the notebook. It's hard to describe what postpartum depression actually feels like. Yet, in this chapter, I attempt to do just that by organizing and sharing the experiences of the women I spoke with, situated within previous studies on the manifestation of postpartum depression.

Postpartum depression manifested in five notable ways for the women I interviewed: extreme anxiety and obsessions, intrusive thoughts of escape, insomnia, feeling overwhelmed, and maternal failure.

Extreme Anxiety and Obsessions

Many of the mothers I interviewed experienced extreme anxiety and obsessions during postpartum depression. For example, I spoke with Katherine,[1] who was convinced she was dying after the birth of her child. Her blood pressure was high, and she knew it was the worst-case scenario. "I just couldn't get it out of my head that I was—I was dying, like that was where I was. I was dying; I was leaving my children." She feared she would die and leave her children abandoned and uncared for.

Katherine did not die, and according to health professionals, her fears were unfounded. She had elevated blood pressure, but her life was not at risk. That didn't stop the extreme anxiety and obsessions over her health, though. If she died, who would care for her baby?

Sometimes, a specific event during the early days of postpartum triggered the obsessive thoughts, like Katherine's experience with high blood pressure. Other mothers described constantly obsessing over and worrying about their child's care, often unable to dismiss thoughts related to catastrophic, yet unlikely, scenarios. Mothers mentioned fearing SIDS (Sudden Infant Death Syndrome), dropping their child, and other potential tragedies. One mother mentioned being scared to take her baby out in the car alone or even leave the house.

While any mother may experience worry or anxiety related to their new baby, for these women, these thoughts were all-encompassing and impacted their day-to-day functioning and well-being. For example, Grace shared that she would "ruminate on those to the point where that's all I could think about, and it was very suffocating, and I couldn't like move beyond those moments."

[1] All participant names are pseudonyms. For participant demographics, see notes on method, found in the Appendix.

Grace's testimony shows how these anxieties and thoughts impacted her daily well-being. Another way mothers identified that they were experiencing a mood disorder was by recognizing their intrusive thoughts.

Intrusive Thoughts of Escape

In addition to anxiety and obsessions related to the life of their child and themselves, mothers spoke of having intrusive thoughts related to harming themselves or taking a step to escape their lives, such as running away or leaving their husbands. The women who shared these thoughts identified them as abnormal and terrifying. These thoughts were intrusive in that they were unwelcome, invasive, and threatening in the women's minds—additionally, these intrusive thoughts related to the mothers escaping themselves or their familial relationships. No individual said outright that they thought about ending their lives. One mother mentioned having a strong urge to hurt herself, but when she realized it was serious, she had her husband take her to the emergency room.

For others, their intrusive thoughts manifested as a way to escape or disappear. For example, one mother said, "I would say things like, 'I just want to go to sleep forever' or 'Just put me down and just let me sleep.' That was basically it, but I think it got—it was more than just like sleep deprivation talk. It was suicidal ideation." Other mothers described thoughts such as thinking their family would be better off without them, feeling that they were making everything worse by being around or wanting to run away. In these situations, individuals did not explicitly have thoughts of ending their lives, but these types of thoughts are related to suicidal thinking or self-destruction.

For other mothers, the intrusive thoughts did not manifest as suicidal ideation or self-harm but as thoughts relating to their relationship with their husbands. For example, one mother mentioned she had thoughts of divorcing her husband while at the same time describing her husband as being very supportive. Another mother mentioned feeling very angry at her husband. Along with these intrusive thoughts, several mothers I spoke with experienced insomnia.

Insomnia

Seven of the women I interviewed described experiencing insomnia. Ellen hadn't slept for months. The insomnia was overwhelming. She dreaded the thought of having to wake up in the middle of the night, dreaded it to the point that it was preventing her from sleeping at all. She told me, "I was not sleeping. I've heard of people saying, like, I haven't slept for months, and now when they say that I'm like, it's a real thing." Even when her baby was sleeping for more extended periods, Ellen's dread prevented her from getting the sleep she desired and critically needed.

Ellen wasn't the only mother I interviewed who mentioned the dread of waking up. Julia said, "I had like dread about going to sleep . . . Because I didn't know when the baby was going to wake up and interrupt that, and I needed that sleep so desperately."[2] Paradoxically, the fact that Julia needed sleep prevented her from getting sleep.

The insomnia these women experienced differed from the sleep loss caused by feeding or caring for their infants. Mothers could not sleep even when their baby was sleeping because of their other postpartum depression symptoms, such as anxiety. Other mothers discussed not being able to sleep even though their child was sleeping through the night or when someone else was responsible for getting up with their child during the night. These challenges with sleep were often related to other anxieties or obsessions mentioned by mothers. Descriptions of postpartum depression do not always mention insomnia; however, the lack of sleep was detrimental to those who experienced it. Along with the physical experience of insomnia, those I spoke with mentioned feeling overwhelmed during postpartum.

2 Ellipses in quotes reflect text removed from the transcript to represent the discussion at hand more clearly.

Overwhelmed

Mothers described feeling extremely overwhelmed during their postpartum depression. For example, Felicity talked about how she felt like she couldn't accomplish anything, saying, "I felt like I was just kind of going through the motions of the day and trying to get from day to day. I didn't feel like I had anything extra to give. Yeah, it felt like just kind of this complete stripping away of anything extra besides survival mode."

Like Felicity, other mothers mentioned feeling like it was taking all they could manage to survive. About half of the mothers mentioned experiences such as "drowning" in tasks, feeling overwhelmed by their responsibilities or day-to-day tasks, and being unable to focus. Isabella said, "I just felt overwhelmed. It was like I was drowning in everything that needed to be accomplished." Other mothers mentioned struggling with accomplishing simple daily tasks, such as making a grocery list. The fact that these women lacked the energy or ability to complete daily tasks exacerbated their feelings of failure, a sentiment that all the women I interviewed mentioned.

Maternal Failure

Ashley told me she felt like she was failing because she wasn't doing the things expected of her, saying:

> You know it brought up a lot of guilt because I wasn't, you know, doing stuff around the house. Or you know, cleaning or taking care of myself. Which I felt like that's what I needed to do now that I wasn't working and I was staying at home. That was my job now, is to maintain a house and to raise a child, and I felt like I was really failing at doing all of that.

Even though she cared for an infant, which is an intense and full-time job, Ashley felt guilty that she couldn't maintain her home or appearance to pre-baby standards. In fact, all the mothers I interviewed experienced feelings of maternal failure during their postpartum depression.

Maternal failure includes feelings such as not being enough, failing, or being a bad mom. Mothers used terms like "failure," "shame," and "guilt" to describe how they felt in the postpartum period. Mothers related these feelings to failing to reach breastfeeding goals, balancing work/home life, not fulfilling their perceived duties in the home, and the fact that they were experiencing depressive symptoms at a time when they felt they should feel happy.

For example, Mimi shared that she told her husband, "I can't do this, and that I'm not a good mom. And I don't know what I'm doing. And that I'm pretty sure the baby hates me." Rather than recognizing that all new mothers struggle when learning how to care for their infant, Mimi felt that she must be a bad mom when she struggled with caring for her infant and soothing his cries. Mimi and Ashley had expectations of what they could accomplish during their postpartum period and felt a sense of failure when they could not meet their own expectations.

At other times, it was the diagnosis of postpartum depression itself that led mothers to feelings of failure. Katherine said that after she was diagnosed, she felt like a failure, saying, "I was failing as a mother, and I was failing [as a] person. And my mind was failing me, and my body was failing me." Maternal failure was the most common manifestation described by the women I spoke with—every mother I talked to experienced feelings of intense failure.

Conclusion

According to Postpartum Support International (PSI, 2024), postpartum depression can manifest in many ways—including but not limited to feelings of anger, crying and sadness, loss of interest or joy, feelings of guilt or hopelessness, physical changes such as appetite or sleep disturbance, and lack of interest in one's child. Furthermore, while there are several specific ways to categorize perinatal mood or anxiety disorders (PMADs), such as postpartum anxiety, Post-Traumatic Stress Disorder, and postpartum obsessive-compulsive disorder, generally speaking, symptoms of these conditions can overlap in a PMAD experience and are more commonly referred to as postpartum depression. Researchers attempting to theorize the experience of postpartum depression have called it "a dangerous thief that robs mothers of the love and happiness they expected to feel toward their newborn babies" (Beck, 2002, p. 453). Indeed, postpartum depression can be debilitating and traumatic for mothers, as shown in the experiences outlined in this chapter.

Nevertheless, postpartum depression remains a stigmatized and poorly understood condition (Elliott et al., 2020). The stereotypes associated with the condition include a desire to harm one's children and/or oneself, perpetuated by media accounts of women harming or killing their children (Holman & McKeever, 2017). These cases, which involve the separate disease of postpartum psychosis, are sometimes mischaracterized as postpartum depression in media reports (Holman & McKeever, 2017). Additionally, news, media, and popular culture often portray women experiencing postpartum depression as not loving their infants and children. Family members, friends, romantic partners, and mothers themselves hold these negative stereotypes.

The women I spoke with described part of their postpartum depression manifestation as extreme anxiety and obsessions. While not always listed as a symptom of postpartum depression specifically, anxiety and obsessive thoughts are conceptualized as part of postpartum depression in theories about the condition (Beck, 2002; Mollard, 2014). PSI (2024) categorizes "constant worry, feeling that something bad is going to happen, and racing thoughts" (np) as anxiety during postpartum. However, a fear of being left alone with the infant and hypervigilance in protecting the infant are categorized as obsessive-compulsive symptoms (PSI, 2024). According to PSI, up to 20 percent of people will experience perinatal anxiety, and 16.9 percent of postpartum mothers will experience obsessive-compulsive symptoms. Additionally, the experiences of anxiety and obsessive thoughts of the women highlighted here align with previous qualitative work on postpartum depression, where researchers identified extreme anxiety and obsessive thinking as key components of postpartum depression (Beck, 1993; Mollard, 2014). Understanding anxiety and obsessive thinking as a core part of the postpartum depression experience can help women, their relational partners, and healthcare providers diagnose and treat the condition.

Second, several women described having intrusive thoughts of escape. Neither Beck (1993) nor Mollard (2014) describes suicidal thoughts as part of the postpartum depression experience. However, more recent work on postpartum depression found that 10.4 percent of Canadian women had thoughts of self-harm during the postpartum period (Palladino et al., 2020). Notably, more than half of the mothers I spoke with shared thoughts about escaping their lives and/or relationships. Perhaps the mothers I interviewed shared these experiences because of their comfort level in talking about their postpartum depression, or perhaps those who experienced these symptoms had more severe levels of postpartum depression. These intrusive thoughts of escape are more in line with common stereotypes surrounding postpartum depression. It may be that these thoughts are common for women experiencing postpartum depression; however, they are often stigmatized, face-threatening, and horrifying to those who experience them and, therefore, less likely to be disclosed. When women have these types of thoughts, it may threaten their identities as mothers.

Along with destructive thoughts, insomnia and feeling overwhelmed are understood to be symptoms of postpartum depression, as defined by PSI (2024). The experiences of feeling significantly overwhelmed or strained align with descriptions of postpartum depression, where women have described "enveloping fogginess" (Beck, 2006, p. 44) that takes over their ability to concentrate.

Finally, research with American mothers makes it clear that one of the main feelings mothers experience in postpartum depression is the failure to fulfill their perception of "mother" (e.g., Abrams & Curran, 2011; Beck, 2002; Mollard, 2014). The notion of maternal failure is prevalent throughout the research on postpartum depression experiences. In their grounded theory study exploring the intersections of postpartum depression, poverty, and motherhood, Abrams and Curran (2011) found mothers felt their postpartum depression, poverty, and single status all contributed to feelings of maternal failure, yet postpartum depression symptoms were more problematic for mothers than poverty when it came to maternal identity formation. In Beck's (2002) meta-synthesis of postpartum depression studies, Beck found that "women held unrealistic expectations of motherhood, which were shattered by the reality of their own lives as new mothers" (p. 470). Beck further articulates that the reality of their experiences led mothers to become overwhelmed, feel like failures, and bear extreme guilt.

Furthermore, mothers who felt this way also felt abnormal in that other mothers did not feel as they did (Beck, 2002). Mollard (2014) identified crushed maternal expectations as the first and essential contributing factor to postpartum depression, writing that after women find that the reality of motherhood does not meet their expectations, "the woman experiences a sense of shame or guilt from being unable to meet her idealized expectation of what motherhood is supposed to be like" (p. 660). The mothers I spoke with and mothers in previous research associated maternal failure with their postpartum depression.

Previous explorations into postpartum depression show that these experiences have identity implications for mothers. Research suggests that mothers experience a "loss of identity" postpartum (Abrams & Curran, 2011; Mollard, 2014; Vik & Hafting, 2012). Indeed, the mothers I interviewed recognized their symptoms as unlike their usual selves. For example, Felicity said, "Yeah, it felt really scary. I felt—I didn't feel like myself at all." Not only was Felicity going through postpartum depression symptoms, but she felt like these symptoms were untrue to her core self. Several women described feeling "out of control" of themselves and their bodies. Mollard (2014) goes as far as to say that "loss of sense of self may be a key component to recognizing postpartum depression as distinct from other regular depressive symptoms" (p. 662). The fact that mothers I spoke to felt they were not in control of who they were or how they functioned clearly presents identity problems.

In addition to a loss of their sense of self, when discussing feelings of failure and other experiences of postpartum depression, mothers mentioned how these feelings were negated, amplified, or even provoked by others. An individual's interactions with others have implications for identity. Women learn how to be mothers not only through experience but also through interactions with other mothers and relational partners. Expectations for how a mother should behave and feel are set through cultural norms and interpersonal interactions. While we know that women who experience postpartum depression have feelings of identity loss and maternal failure, we can better understand how these identity problems and feelings of failure manifest, the role of others in these experiences, and how cultural norms and ideals can manifest in everyday interactions through using CTI as a sensitizing framework to explore identity. Exploring identity manifestations and tensions with CTI offers a way to separate and investigate influences on identity by considering identity as layers. In the following several chapters, I use the framework of CTI to explain women's identity manifestations and tensions as they experienced postpartum depression.

Chapter Summary

The mothers I interviewed experienced extreme anxiety and obsessions, where they ruminated on an unlikely scenario to the point it affected their daily functioning and well-being; intrusive thoughts of escape, where they had unwelcomed and scary thoughts of escaping their lives; insomnia; and a sense of feeling extremely overwhelmed from the daily responsibilities and tasks they faced. The unifying experience of every mother I interviewed was the intense and overwhelming feelings of maternal failure, shame, and guilt, which aligns with previous research exploring experiences of postpartum depression. Mothers mentioned how they didn't feel like themselves and how others influenced their feelings; these experiences, along with the feelings of maternal failure, point to a need to understand identity tensions women face during postpartum depression.

2

The Changing Self—Personal Identity amid Mothering and Postpartum Depression

Ellen had always wanted to be a mom, telling me, "Growing up, I always thought career-wise, I was going to be a mom. Like I was going to stay at home with my kids, and I'm going to love it." However, after she had her first child, she didn't experience the instant feelings of connection and love that she had thought she would, considering how this was something she had always wanted. "That made me very sad. It's kind of torture, like taking care of this little person that I have no desire to take care of and no connection to." On top of that, Ellen felt like she had lost herself, saying, "I was empty. I was like a shell of myself. Just a little shell of my former self. I wasn't really in there." She felt as if she couldn't control herself. She wept all the time. She didn't know who to trust, including herself. These feelings—the loss of self, the expectation that she would love being a mom, and then not feeling that instant connection—left her devastated.

In this chapter, I explore how mothers described themselves in the context of postpartum depression, with attention to how their personal identities shifted, fragmented, or were redefined. Importantly, for women in this study, the postpartum experience is the experience of postpartum depression; the two are inseparable and together shape maternal identity.

I conceptualize these experiences using CTI as a sensitizing theory, and my focus here is on the personal layer of identity. The personal layer of identity refers to the individual and encompasses constructs such as self-concept and self-image (Hecht et al., 2005). For example, one might consider oneself an "empathetic person." The personal layer of identity was conceptualized based on psychological research into self and personality and can be associated with individualism (Hecht, 2015). Personal identity can also be self-evaluation

(Wagner et al., 2016) and the social identity labels with which one identifies (Hecht, 2015).

First, I share three broad conclusions regarding the manifestation of the personal layer of identity: women felt like they had become a different person, women drew on their salient social identities to contextualize their pre- and post-natal experience, and some used their mood disorder diagnosis to understand their symptoms as different from permanent changes in their personalities. Next, I discuss the identity gap women faced as they struggled to fit their self-identity into their new role as mothers. Finally, I share how the experience of postpartum depression had lasting impacts on personal identity for women and discuss the implications of my analysis for the personal layer of CTI.

Personal Layer Themes and Gaps

"The Person I Became"

After she had her child, Ellen felt like she had become a shell of her former self. Ellen's experience is common—mothers feel like they become a different person when they experience postpartum depression. When I experienced postpartum depression, I didn't understand that my symptoms were temporary. I knew I was a different person, but I felt like that was just who I was now, and I was going to have to learn to live with this miserable person I now called "me" and do the best I could to try to hide that miserable part from those I loved.

The mothers I interviewed described themselves in a way that was foreign to their core selves. Descriptions from mothers included negative feelings and self-evaluations that influenced perceptions of self. For example, Grace said, "I usually don't cry very much whatsoever. But it just, that's kind of the person I became . . . constantly upset, constantly crying." Here, Grace compares how she perceives her previous self to how she was while experiencing postpartum depression. Other mothers used words such as empty, sad, lost, and devastated to describe themselves during the time they were experiencing postpartum depression. Similarly, Hannah said, "I almost didn't know who I was anymore." These descriptions point to a dislocation of the self, a feeling of both losing who they were and becoming someone they did not recognize or want to be.

Drawing on Social Identities

In addition to describing how they changed in self-concept and self-evaluation as they experienced postpartum depression, some women shared various social identities with which they self-identified and how they used those identities to make sense of their postpartum depression. Hecht (2015) situates the social identities that a person considers part of their self-concept as part of the personal layer of identity. The mothers who drew on social identities discussed racial and cognitive identities in relation to themselves.

Both women I interviewed who identified racially as Black referenced their identity as a Black woman as part of their experience with postpartum depression, especially concerning their experience within the healthcare system. Dawn said, "I think that being a Black mom makes a huge difference in my experience. And um, like being able to trust doctors." Additionally, Maria discussed how being Black made it harder for her to find mental health providers that she trusted and that validated her experience. Knowing that Black women are at an increased risk for postpartum depression (Bauman et al., 2020) and that Black women are less likely to receive adequate mental health care after the delivery of their child (Kozhimannil et al., 2011), this may have heightened the salience of race for Dawn and Maria as they interacted with healthcare providers during their pregnancy and postpartum.

Along with racial identity, mothers drew on other labels to understand their experiences. Julia shared how she and other members of her family were recently diagnosed with a bio-neurological developmental disability. She linked her identity as a person with this condition to her parenting experiences, especially concerning anxiety, breastfeeding, and childbirth. In addition to developmental conditions, some mothers also described how mood disorders shaped their sense of self.

Identifying as Someone with a Mood Disorder

Finally, within the personal layer of identity, some mothers reflected on their experience with mood disorders. By considering the symptoms as part of the diagnosis rather than as part of their personality, these mothers were able to situate their experience within their self-identity without the threat to their self. Ellen shared this with me when she said, "You are not your intrusive thoughts. They are a symptom of depression. They're disturbing because they are not you." More than half of the mothers I interviewed had a history of mood disorders before their experience with postpartum depression, and some drew on their identity as a person with anxiety, depression, or other mood disorders to understand their symptoms as part of a mood disorder, not as part of their personalities. Interestingly, for some, like Cierra, the diagnosis of postpartum depression helped her separate her mood disorder from herself, saying, "It's interesting because I felt for the first like 20 years of my life everything about my identity was totally wrapped up in anxiety because it drove everything that I did and every choice that I made." Like others, Cierra shared how, before her postpartum depression diagnosis, she had incorporated her anxiety as part of her sense of self instead of as a symptom of a mood disorder. Other women also shared how they had dealt with anxiety since they were a child or had been on antidepressant medications before becoming pregnant. Perhaps because these mothers had previously dealt with a mood disorder, the fact of being diagnosed with postpartum depression was not necessarily detrimental to their sense of self or self-identity.

Mothers did not necessarily relate the diagnosis of postpartum depression to maternal failure. In most cases, the sense of failure and shame was related to the behaviors and feelings that manifested as part of postpartum depression, not to the diagnosis. Nevertheless, this was not always the case (such as when Katherine described how, after learning she had postpartum depression, she felt her body and her mind were failing her). One factor that may have influenced the women's self-perception is the fact that I recruited mainly through postpartum support groups. Postpartum depression is more likely to be validated and normalized within these groups; therefore, those with whom I spoke may have already dealt with any issues of self-stigma related to their postpartum depression diagnosis by the time they conversed with me.

Additionally, those who feel a strong self-stigma of the postpartum depression label are unlikely to agree to be interviewed, making it improbable that I would interview mothers who would convey this. It may be that the symptoms of postpartum depression are what is stigmatizing to mothers rather than the diagnosis. In addition to the ways the personal layer of identity manifested for mothers, they also described tensions between their personal layer and other layers of identity. One tension women experienced was not feeling like a "mother."

Personal-Relational Gap: Not Feeling like a "Mother"

As mentioned in the opening paragraph, Ellen didn't experience the instant connection she had expected when her son was born. Mothers experienced a personal-relational identity gap when they did not immediately internalize the role identity of "mother." The identity gap led to a feeling of guilt that they did not feel an instant connection with their child. For example, Mimi, whose child was only weeks old at the time of the interview, talked about how she did not yet identify with the label of "mother," saying, "Like I know he is my son, and I know that he came from me obviously, and I know that he is my responsibility, but I don't know, I thought you would just feel like a mom immediately. But I just kind of feel like I take care of this tiny human." Mimi thought she would develop a relational identity with her infant immediately but recognized that she had not yet taken in this role and her relationship with her infant as part of her self-identity. Similarly, Ashley described not feeling an instant connection with her infant, saying,

> When he was born, and they put him on my chest, I didn't get that big rush. I was tired. I was scared. I was, you know, nervous. Overwhelmed. And I felt really guilty for that. 'Cause I didn't get that feeling, and it made me feel like maybe I didn't love him the way that other mothers love their children.

Ashley shares the idea that "other mothers" have an instant love and connection with their children, describing not only her personal and relational layers and how they were in conflict but also calling on a communal identity of mother.

Ellen and Mimi referenced ideas about how a mother's instinct and connection to one's child should be immediate and natural. So, while this gap was related to women's personal selves and their relationship with their infants, expectations of motherhood, conveyed through both macro and micro messages, influenced feelings of guilt and shame when a woman did not immediately feel like a mother.

Lasting Impacts

I also was interested in exploring what lasting effects postpartum depression had on identity. Berquist et al. (2019) found in their study of refugee experiences that temporary identities can be temporary for some individuals while remaining more lasting for others, even when they are no longer a primary identity. Therefore, it makes sense that the temporal experience of postpartum depression may have lasting identity impacts.

Positive Long-Term Impact on Self

More prominent than any negatively veiled lasting impacts of postpartum depression were the positive impacts mentioned by women. Ellen described herself as "more vulnerable," "more open," and "more spontaneous"; experiencing postpartum depression changed her sense of self in positive ways. Similarly, Eva mentioned being more empathetic in that by going through this experience, she was now able to understand other mothers and other people in general who were having mental health issues or struggling. Dawn talked about how, by going through postpartum depression, she learned to prioritize herself more and understand the importance of her mental health. Overall, these women felt that they were able to grow in positive ways by going through postpartum depression.

Continued Mental Health Impacts

Some women continued to experience anxiety and depression beyond the postpartum period. While these women connected their episodes to postpartum depression, healthcare professionals told them that it was no longer postpartum depression. For example, Katherine shared that healthcare professionals told her she no longer had postpartum depression, saying:

> At a certain point, they just tell you it's no longer postpartum. You just have generalized anxiety now. Your hormones should have settled out. You know it's not this anymore; I mean to the point that my therapist told me that. She's like the postpartum is gone; like you just have generalized anxiety. I don't really know how much more I can help you.

Katherine's postpartum depression diagnosis was taken away from her by her therapist after the postpartum period, and her therapist even went as far as to say she could no longer help Katherine with managing her anxiety. Isabella talked about how she was continuing to use medication and therapy at eighteen months postpartum, saying:

> So it's like not even, you know, postpartum anymore. I guess it's just who I am. And that makes—that's kind of a hard, like a hard thing to live with. Like you know, it's not just like your hormones, or it's not just postpartum depression anymore; it's just part of who you are now. And that makes me kind of bummed out.

Like Katherine, Isabella refers to hormones, linking postpartum depression with hormonal imbalances; however, voicing her opinion that once the postpartum period is over, the symptoms are no longer postpartum depression, which is a temporary illness, but who she has become. In both cases, these women felt that their mental health diagnosis had become part of who they were; unlike postpartum depression, this was a lasting diagnosis. While these women struggled with their ongoing mental health diagnosis related to their identity, others talked about continuing treatment in a more positive way. For example, Cierra said, "I've been taking Zoloft ever since my son was born, so I've been taking it for eight years now, and I don't plan on stopping. I feel like it would have changed my life back in high school had I been on it before." Cierra did not see the medication as a threat to her identity. Instead, she appreciated the positive effect it had on her life. Cierra had suffered from anxiety her whole life and felt that her postpartum depression experience enabled her to get the treatment she needed.

Conclusion

It took Ellen a "solid 18 months" to come out of the "pits of PPD" and feel like she had a good bond with her child. She told me that she felt more engaged, more loving, and more concerned. "I've learned a lot of lessons going through postpartum depression, and I'm sure I'm going to have a lot more lessons to come as [child] grows up." For Ellen, her postpartum depression had immediate adverse impacts on her personal identity—she felt like a different person, and she felt a gap in identity when her expectations of what it would feel like to be a mother didn't match up with what she experienced. But Ellen's postpartum depression had mixed long-term impacts—such as growing as a person and influencing her choice of having more children. Ellen's experience mirrors that of many of the mothers with whom I spoke.

Mothers experiencing postpartum depression feel an impact on their personal identities. The mothers I interviewed felt that they became a different person than their usual selves, typically a person who experienced negative feelings such as sadness, emptiness, or desperation. Some expressed how their salient social identities influenced their postpartum depression experience in unique ways, and others used their postpartum depression diagnosis as a way to reconcile their feelings and behavior with their personal identity. I identified an identity gap between the personal and relational layers when mothers had expectations of what motherhood would be like, and then their lived experiences did not meet these expectations. Postpartum depression had a lasting effect on the sense of self for mothers—most felt they were changed positively; however, some continued to face mental health challenges.

We know that women feel a loss of self as they become mothers and/or experience postpartum depression (Abrams & Curran, 2011; Beck, 2002;

Cronin-Fisher & Parcell, 2019; Mollard, 2014; Vik & Hafting, 2012); the testimonies here support this conception of a loss of self as something inherent to the postpartum period. The fact that these women felt they became a different person aligns with previous research exploring women's experiences of postpartum depression, where mothers feel an identity loss as they struggle with the loss of previous identities and as mothers must construct a new self as they make sense of their permanent life changes (Abrams & Curran, 2011). This process of identity reconstruction is further shaped by the salience of various social identities, which may become particularly prominent in the context of postpartum depression.

Our various social identities become more salient based on how we perceive ourselves as different or similar to others in a particular context (Greenaway et al., 2018). When mothers saw themselves as having different social identities (racial, cognitive), those identities became salient to their experience, which was reinforced by their interactions with others. For example, none of the mothers who identified as white mentioned their whiteness as a factor in their postpartum depression experience. The personal identity frame was salient for Dawn and Maria as they made sense of their experiences based on their personal identity as Black women, and for Julia, as she made sense of her experience through her identity as a person with a cognitive disability. Another identity discussed in the personal layer was identifying as someone with a mood disorder. Researchers have connected postpartum depression to social identity before; Seymour-Smith et al. (2017) found that mothers who experienced social identity loss through loss of group memberships were more likely to experience postpartum depression.

The stigma of a postpartum depression diagnosis was not an overwhelming concern for the women I spoke with, likely because most were involved in some sort of maternal mental health support advocacy initiative. Furthermore, a diagnosis of an illness can help individuals understand their symptoms as something external to their true selves rather than a permanent part of themselves (Palmer-Wackerly et al., 2018), which aligns with previous findings of maternal failure as part of postpartum depression, where postpartum depression symptoms were what caused mothers to feel failure, not the diagnosis itself (Abrams & Curran, 2011; Mollard, 2014). Indeed, women who think their postpartum depression symptoms are a sign of bad motherhood rather than a mental health illness report feeling shame and isolating themselves (Mollard, 2014).

The personal-relational identity gap reflects broader cultural scripts that assume maternal instinct and instant connection (Rowe & Fisher, 2015; Scharp & Thomas, 2017), contributing to feelings of guilt when the experience doesn't match expectations. However, women do not always feel an instant bond with their infants, and mothering is a learned experience (Scharp & Thomas, 2017).

As individuals experience identity gaps, they engage in identity negotiation processes, where these gaps are mitigated or individuals learn to cope with them. Over time, gaps may become no longer negative for individuals (Maeda & Hecht, 2012). While postpartum depression as a medical diagnosis ends after twelve months postpartum, women may continue to have depressive symptoms beyond that timeframe. In their study of postpartum women, McMahon et al. (2008) found that more than half the women diagnosed with postpartum depression continued to experience episodes of depression beyond twelve months postpartum.

While this chapter explored how women experience identity changes internally, the next chapter will examine how those identities are performed and enacted in communication with others—how postpartum depression affects the ways mothers present themselves and interact with the world around them.

Chapter Summary

Mothers felt like they became a different person as they experienced postpartum depression, losing who they used to be and having that self replaced with a new person they did not want to be. Some mothers felt their salient social identities impacted their experience with postpartum depression, specifically, racial identity and cognitive identity were important sense-makers for a few of the women with whom I spoke. These identities were salient because they saw themselves as different than the majority. For some women, their history of mood disorders was a salient part of their self-identity and served as a sense-making factor when they situated their identities within their postpartum depression experience, although all women who had a history of mood disorders expressed the notable differences between their previous experiences and postpartum depression. Mothers experienced a personal-relational identity gap when their personal identity did not align with the role identity of "mother." Women reported expecting to feel an instant connection to their child or an instant maternal feeling, and when that connection or feeling did not manifest, they thought something must be wrong with them as a person. Despite the negative experiences of postpartum depression, many mothers I spoke with mentioned that this challenging time left a positive impact on their lives, describing themselves as being more empathic or more open. Some mothers spoke about how they have continued mental health challenges, despite being out of the postpartum period.

3

The Enacted Self—Enacting Motherhood and Postpartum Depression

Isabella had an inter-dwelling catheter, or as she called it, a "pee bag," attached to her for a week after she delivered. "I had a catheter for seven days. It was awful," she recalled. Her labor went so fast that she couldn't receive an epidural. Then, after she delivered, she couldn't empty her bladder. The doctors told her the rapid descent of her daughter had affected her bladder, bruising the backside. The delivery and the aftermath left her body feeling broken. And now she had an infant to care for.

In addition to her bladder problems, Isabella had trouble breastfeeding. It was hard for her to get enough milk. She describes feeling physically inadequate. "They're like looking at your nipples, and they want it to look like this. And you're like, I don't have that. And they're like, 'Because of your shallow nipples.' I was like, no one ever told me that I have shallow nipples." The lactation consultants labeled Isabella's body as inadequate, which left her with a feeling of failure.

Isabella spent the first week at home in pain, self-conscious of her catheter, and struggling to make enough milk to feed her infant. The lactation consultants she saw were adamant that she breastfeed only and not use formula as a supplement. She felt a lack of support, felt embarrassed to ask for support due to her condition, and felt like she wasn't mothering in the right way.

Isabella's experience represents a tension between how she enacted mothering and how others told her she should enact mothering. Instead of telling her she deserved and should seek help in feeding her infant during the first few weeks so her body could heal, healthcare professionals pushed her to breastfeed exclusively. "I needed real physical support," she recalled. I share Isabella's experience to highlight several aspects of enacted identity, especially the tension mothers faced as they enacted motherhood in a way that didn't align with societal or medical mandates.

Social behavior is the enacted identity or the enacted layer of identity. In the enacted layer of identity, the self is seen as a performance. If a person identifies as an empathetic individual, do they exhibit empathy in their interactions with others? What behaviors and communication practices do they use to enact empathy? Foundations of this layer of identity come from sociology and the idea of the "performed self" (Hecht, 2015). Indeed, Goffman's (1959) dramaturgical theory of identity fits well with this aspect of CTI. Hecht (2015) writes, "CTI agrees with Goffman that even though all communication does not enact identity and identity is more than just communication, when we talk we *are* our identities" (p. 180). CTI looks at communication as it expresses identity.

Importantly, the enacted layer of identity is difficult to separate from the relational layer because when a person presents a self through communication to another, they usually have a goal of wanting that other to accept their presentation (Goffman, 1959; Jung, 2011). Indeed, in expanding Goffman's Facework Theory, researchers have argued that individuals perform a self in relation to others (McBride, 2018). Therefore, while I discuss enacted identity here, it is essential to remember that an enacted identity is always enacted in relation to another. I naturally refer to relational others when describing mothers' enacted identity behaviors.

Enactment Behavior—Seeking Treatment

Not as prominent as other themes, but still noteworthy, was how mothers related their actions in seeking treatment for postpartum depression to their identity. For example, Cierra said:

> I'm kind of a type A person, so I was like, let's just do all these things. I will go to a counselor. I will talk to my OB, and I'll look up a support group and . . . Because I have like background in studying mental health, and it's always

> been important to me. I'm like, there's no weirdness there. I was like, yeah, I'll just do all the things.

Here, Cierra relates her self-concept to the actions she took to seek treatment for her postpartum depression, identifying herself as a "Type-A" person and saying that because of that and her background, she decided to "do all the things" in treating her postpartum depression. Indeed, individuals who understand their illness as a temporary part of their overall personal identity can seek treatment quickly (Palmer-Wackerly et al., 2018).

Hannah discussed how she sought treatment for her postpartum depression before disclosing it to her husband, saying, "So I felt like if it wasn't just coming from me at home one evening, and it was like OK, I've talked to a doctor I've, you know, been prescribed this, and I've been referred to this, I feel like then he had more open ears." She relates her enacted practices of seeking a postpartum depression diagnosis to her relational identity, saying that she felt her husband would be more receptive to her claims of postpartum depression (hence, her identity performance of someone with postpartum depression) if she already received a diagnosis from her doctor confirming that these symptoms were due to an illness, not just a changing part of herself.

In addition to seeking postpartum depression treatment, some mothers described how they did not seek treatment. For example, Hannah mentioned how, at first, she didn't feel comfortable calling her doctor's office to ask about postpartum depression, so she called to ask about something else and then casually brought up postpartum depression. Similarly, Ashley said, "I still think it's that kind of . . . that feeling of shame where you don't really want to reach out for the help because you want to be able to figure it out on your own, or you either just don't know how to express what's going on." In this case, the perceived effectiveness of their disclosure seems to have influenced their choices (Choi et al., 2016). Both Ashley and Hannah discussed not seeking treatment initially because they didn't know how to communicate what was happening to them.

Mothers' postpartum depression manifested within their enacted layer of identity in how they approached seeking treatment. Mothers experienced tensions in their enacted identity when another individual negated their performance of motherhood.

Enacted-Relational Gap: Mothering Wrong

As mentioned in the opening story, Isabella's postnatal team gave very specific instructions on how to feed her daughter. She told me, "The lactation consultants really, really forced some, I would say, not evidence-based information about breastfeeding onto us and really kind of choked it down our throats." She also told me how she received "unsolicited" and "not helpful" advice from her mother, her siblings, and even people she hadn't talked to in years who reached out via social media. She recalled how people "all of a sudden have different opinions than me, and they feel like that it's their calling to share their opinion [on child-rearing]."

I describe this communication problem as an enacted-relational gap, where a woman's enacted identity as a mother was not aligned with the ascribed identity from others. Most of the messages creating gaps in this instance were related to breastfeeding. A lactation consultant told Julia that the way she delivered, something she had no control over, would affect her ability to breastfeed her child. Julia told me, "I also had a lactation consultant make me feel bad about, you know, the way I delivered because she said that impacted the nursing." The lactation consultant identified Julia as someone unable to breastfeed. Also related to feeding, healthcare professionals told Bethany that she wasn't giving her infant enough breastmilk and had to stay in the hospital. She recollected them saying, "'Oh like, he just has these hunger cries. You guys have to stay another day.' And so it, the whole breastfeeding thing, especially in a hospital, was very not helpful. It made me feel like I was failing." Bethany was trying to enact an identity of a good mother by breastfeeding, but the hospital staff did not confirm that identity.

Additionally, a lactation consultant later told Bethany that she should commit to exclusive breastfeeding, even after she mentioned her mental health struggles and how getting support from others through bottle feeding her child would help her mentally. Again, health professionals advised Bethany to change her parenting approach without considering the impact on her own health. Similarly, healthcare professionals advised Ellen that while she was at home with her infant, she should not pump breast milk and feed it from a bottle; rather, the "best" way to feed her child was directly from the breast. Even though both these women were giving their children breastmilk, that was not enough for healthcare professionals; they told both women they should be feeding from the breast to do the best for their child.

In the long term, mothers continued to call upon their postpartum depression experience in their enactments by becoming advocates for postpartum women and through the decision not to have more children.

Lasting Impacts

Becoming an Advocate

Many women discussed feeling a calling to advocate for future mothers who may go through postpartum depression and mothers in general. Most individuals were involved in some sort of volunteer role with a postpartum support organization. Some women felt a calling to give back to the organization because of the help and support they had from volunteer mothers. Dawn, discussing her involvement with a postpartum support organization, said, "I told them I'll do anything for them," reflecting on her commitment to the organization and to helping other mothers.

For a few mothers, the desire to support mothers went beyond a volunteer role. Ellen decided to go back to school to become a counselor, saying, "I want to work with women who have postpartum depression . . . So it's going to stick with me through my career. Yeah, through my career choices and career changes, it's impacted me that much." After her experience, Ellen wanted to focus her career on helping other women. Felicity, who already worked in mental health, also mentioned that she decided to specialize in postpartum mental health after her experience with postpartum depression and went through training to get certified in the postpartum specialty.

Other mothers shared that they felt a desire to normalize the experience of postpartum depression by doing small things, like posting on social media, being open about their experience, or participating in studies such as this one. It makes sense that all mothers in this study would express a desire to normalize the experience of postpartum depression, based on how I recruited women and the fact that those interested in participating in these types of studies have a goal associated with participating—especially as I offered no incentive for participating.

Done Having Children

An additional lasting impact of postpartum depression was that some women said they no longer wanted to have additional children. As framed by those who expressed it, this was a lasting adverse effect. "It's definitely, unfortunately, made us reconsider having more children," said Isabella. Later on, she echoed this lasting impact, saying, "I initially would have wanted a large family."

Eva said, "I think we would have had more kids if I didn't have this experience . . . I hope I don't regret that later on." Eva reflected on how her postpartum depression impacted the joint decision with her husband to be done having children. However, she worried about regretting that decision. Similarly, Ellen said her experience has affected her, as she does not want to have another child, saying, "I know things can change, but I have a pretty strong belief that I'm done." Ellen, like other women, discussed how her postpartum depression impacted her decision to have more children; after this experience, they decided against having additional children. This is a lasting identity impact; women envisioned themselves as a person who would have a certain number of children, and after experiencing postpartum depression, this idea of themselves changed.

However, less than half of the women I spoke with mentioned this as a lasting effect of their postpartum depression. Cierra talked about how her opinion on the number of children she wanted to have started large, then after she had postpartum depression with her first, went to one, but then changed again, and she ended up having another child. She shared advice for other mothers, saying, "If you're in the middle of symptoms, you do not need to make big decisions like that now. And if you change your mind, it's OK." Some mothers felt that this was a permanent impact of their postpartum depression experience. However, as Cierra said, a person or a couple can change their mind.

Conclusion

The enacted layer of identity manifested as women chose whether and how to seek treatment. At times, mothers experienced an enacted-relational identity gap when they were made to feel as if they were not performing the correct actions of mothering by others. Finally, mothers mentioned that their experiences with postpartum depression led them to pursue ways to advocate for postpartum women and sometimes even influenced their choices to have more children.

This relationship between disclosure, social judgment, and advocacy highlights how treatment-seeking behavior becomes a key performance of identity for many mothers navigating postpartum depression. There are barriers to seeking treatment, including views about postpartum depression and negative views of the self with postpartum depression (Hadfield & Wittkowski, 2017). Indeed, fear of being labeled a bad mother can prevent mothers from seeking help or treatment for postpartum depression (Beck, 2002), which is slightly different from fear of being diagnosed with postpartum depression. Mothers negotiated these barriers by drawing on their personal identity (e.g., Type-A person) and taking steps to ensure relational partners' acceptance of their diagnosis. Finally, some mothers had trouble seeking treatment and referenced these barriers as to why they were unable to seek help.

I examined how mothers received messages from others, including healthcare providers and online influencers, telling them that something they were doing as a mother was inadequate or "not right." In their book *You're Doing It Wrong: Mothering, Media, and Medical Expertise*, Johnson and Quinlan (2019) explore the intersections of power, medical expertise, and lay knowledge on social media in the construction of "good" motherhood. Gaps manifested when others told mothers their actions were negatively impacting their child, most commonly concerning breastfeeding. Johnson and Quinlan (2019) discuss the concept of the "expert gaze," in which healthcare experts critique and discipline female bodies and mothering practices—something evident in the experiences I heard.

Furthermore, women are expected to put their child's needs above their own, both in pregnancy and postpartum. However, in other aspects of life, we are told to "put our oxygen mask on first" before helping others. Instead of putting on their oxygen masks first, mothers are expected to put on their children's oxygen masks while they, the mothers, slowly suffocate. These types of messages from others can create identity gaps in mothers experiencing postpartum depression when they are unable to perform mothering practices to the recommended standard and need to take care of their own needs to survive.

This struggle between societal expectations and personal limitations contributes not only to enacted-relational identity gaps but also motivates some mothers to challenge dominant discourses about motherhood altogether. Similarly, in other parenting contexts, individuals and groups have become advocates for promoting alternative discourses surrounding events such as infant loss. For example, the Now I Lay Me Down to Sleep Remembrance Walk enables participants to acknowledge and make visible baby loss rather than silencing infant loss (Willer et al., 2020). Taken together, these experiences demonstrate how postpartum women actively negotiate, resist, and reframe dominant messages about motherhood through communicative acts, ultimately enacting identities that make space for both their struggles and their strengths.

Chapter Summary

Mothers related their decisions to disclose and seek treatment to their identities, with some choosing to disclose and seek treatment right away because they did not perceive the diagnosis as an identity threat. In contrast, others chose not to disclose because they felt they would not be able to communicate effectively what was happening to them. Some mothers experienced an enacted-relational identity gap when they were told they were not enacting motherhood in the "right" way; most of these experiences were related to breastfeeding. Experiencing postpartum depression had lasting impacts on the enacted layer of identity. Mothers discussed their choice to become advocates for new mothers and women experiencing postpartum depression and their choice to have or not have more children due to their experience with postpartum depression.

4

The Collective Self—Communal Identity of a Postpartum Mother

Throughout my interview with Hannah, her reflections revealed how powerfully societal expectations shape women's visions of motherhood, even before they become mothers. "I definitely had some expectations becoming a mother," she told me. She continued, saying:

> Like I thought I was gonna have this baby and I was going to work full time and I was going to have dinner made when I came home, and I was going to have all the laundry done, and this baby was going to start reading by three months old, you know? Like, I thought I was going to have all this stuff done. . . . I feel like that's what women are expected to do now.

As I spoke with Hannah, she described the pressure many women feel as they become mothers, saying, "All of these pressures we have around us to have, you know, this perfect nursery kept ready for a picture to be taken by a photographer at any moment . . . And also have these Pinterest-ready meals ready every night; like the expectation of all of these things, it's just insane."

Hannah's description of "what women are expected to do now" points to the communal identity of a mother. Communal identity is the most challenging layer of CTI to explain because of Western ideas about identity and self (Hecht, 2015). This layer is derived from the ethnographic and cultural study tradition. Western culture associates identity with something that lies within the individual; however, CTI incorporates Confucian philosophical ideas of the self, where the self is part of a collective and individuality is de-emphasized (Hecht et al., 2005). Additionally, CTI incorporates group-based identities and social roles as important aspects of identity, both in how those are internalized in the self and ascribed by others (Hecht et al., 2005).

There is some discrepancy when describing the communal layer of identity. While Hecht frames the communal layer as a macro-level discourse, other scholars have conceptualized the communal layer as how macro-level discourses affect the individual. For example, Soliz and Colaner (2018) write that communal identity "attends to the manner in which larger social discourses . . . and social identities . . . shape how we view ourselves in relation to social expectations and depictions" (p. 81). Another way to think about the communal layer is to say that it recognizes that identities emerge from group memberships. Individuals understand their identity within group memberships and the expectations and stereotypes that go along with those groups (Bergquist et al., 2019). These expectations and stereotypes come from the broader culture. Within the communal layer, one might look at how a culture or society defines "mother," and/or a mother might consider how she "measures up" to the social expectations and depictions of "mother" in her culture.

For my purposes in describing this layer, I recount how the women I spoke with identified a general, imagined identity of "mother" based on societal representations and then discuss the identity gap women faced as they viewed their maternal selves in comparison to this communal identity. Then, I discuss the implications of this ideal of a postpartum mother for the lived experience of mothers with postpartum depression.

Delivery and Recovery Expectations

While actual delivery experiences varied, women shared a common narrative of what they expected to happen during the delivery of their child. For example, Dawn said, "I feel like society tells us that, you know, motherhood is such a beautiful thing, and as soon as you have a baby, you're in your white gown and in the hospital, and you know you're walking around holding your baby, and everything is so perfect."

The use of "society tells you" shows how this conceptualization of post-birth represents a shared cultural ideal rather than something held by Dawn alone. Additionally, Annisa shared how she expected to have an easy delivery because she had taken steps to prepare, saying, "I had a dream that I can deliver normally. You know I did exercise and everything. Ate healthy foods, like I did everything to be able to deliver normally." For Annisa, being able to deliver her child through vaginal birth was part of being a good mother, and therefore she took steps to be able to fit into that identity; however, the way one delivers is usually out of one's control. Other mothers mentioned their delivery, hospital, and recovery experience in relation to the challenges they faced and how it impacted their view of self. Additionally, society expects mothers to have an instant and natural bond with their infant after they deliver their child.

"Natural" and Instant Connection with Child

One idea the women I spoke with shared about becoming a mother was that they would feel an instant love for their child. For example, Ashley said:

> When I was pregnant, I was always told, you know—I had a rough pregnancy—but I was always told, you know, listen, once you have your baby boy and you hold him, everything goes away. It's, you know, it's the best feeling. You get this huge rush of love and emotion, and you know nothing else matters. You don't even remember the pregnancy or the birth.

Ashley experienced a challenging pregnancy, and others helped her maintain the face of a "good mother" by telling her that even though she did not enjoy pregnancy, she would enjoy meeting her newborn son. Ellen also discussed the expectation of feeling immediate love and joy after birth, saying, "You know, once you have your baby, it's uh, rainbows and unicorns . . . Yeah, there's a lot of expectations and pressures that moms . . . they're in love immediately."

These ideas align with ideologies perpetuated by twentieth-century psychology and child development research, which suggest that women biologically desire a child and, when that need is met, will experience joy (Glenn, 1994). While most believed they would form an instant bond with their child after birth, based on their new identity as mothers, some of the women in my study specifically mentioned not feeling an immediate connection with their child. There were also ideas about breastfeeding inherent in women's expectations of mothering.

Breastfeeding Expectations

The women I interviewed linked the desire and ability to breastfeed to the communal postpartum mother identity. For example, Cierra said,

> I think like on top of, on top of your personal beliefs, you have society telling you everything about what you need to do for your kid that is good or right or healthy, and like everyone is telling you that you have to breastfeed. It's the only best way your child is going to get the antibodies that they need, and there's no other way they can get it from you but *from* you.

Here, Cierra discussed how, in addition to the personal desire to provide the best care for one's child through feeding practices, society also sends a strong message about the "best" way to feed infants.

Additionally, some women discussed how "breastfeeding" was defined by practitioners not as feeding the infant breast milk but as feeding the infant from the breast. Ellen, who wanted to pump some breastmilk, was told by a healthcare provider that pumping was not the best mothering practice, remembering, "It was breast. You know, if you're home, if you are home and you're not at work, breast. We'll talk about pumping and storing when you go back to work. That was it." Indeed, a common idea was that "we're all expected to breastfeed," which manifested as part of the communal identity of postpartum mother.

Breastfeeding messages have been shown to have implications for maternal identity based on whether or not mothers feel the messages they have received regarding breastfeeding align with their experience (Hosek et al., 2021). The women who spoke with me felt that to fit in with the communal identity of mother, they were supposed to want to breastfeed their children and do so successfully. Furthermore, mothers recalled a learned expectation that they were supposed to find true joy in motherhood.

Joy and Fulfillment in Mothering

One expectation of postpartum mothering was that, while motherhood was challenging, the joy one feels as a mother would compensate for the difficulty of mothering, and that being a mother was the most important and fulfilling role for a woman. For example, Felicity shared, "I think the messaging that I've received is kind of that you're supposed to enjoy every moment and that there might be hard points, but . . ." Felicity was taught that as a mother, she should enjoy "every moment." Similarly, Julia said one of the prominent ideas she hears about motherhood is that it's hard but the best job, saying, "'It's hard, but it's best job in the world,' is what they say." As mothers absorb societal ideals and messages, incorporating them into their expectations of what motherhood will be like, they often believe they will experience overwhelming joy and fulfillment from mothering.

In addition to receiving messages that motherhood is joyful, women received messages that motherhood should be fulfilling. Julia shared a message she received from a friend, saying, "You know my one girlfriend has a son a year older than mine. I mean, she told it to me, right? It puts your priorities in order. And very suddenly, you know, our lives are ruled by our work, and very suddenly, work doesn't really matter anymore. I mean, it does, but." Here, the idea is that mothering is perhaps not the only job one has; however, it is the most fulfilling job and is the top priority for women. Mothers were also taught that they would be able to "do it all" when it came to mothering.

Moms Can "Do It All"

Finally, women shared the idea that mothers can "do it all," a sentiment reflected in common tropes about mothers, such as "supermom." As mentioned in the chapter opening, Hannah reflected on how mothers are not only expected to care for their children but also to maintain a well-kept and aesthetically pleasing home, prepare homemade meals for their families, and be successful in their careers. Julia shared that she thought, "I want to work, and I want to have a kid. I should be able to do both. Lots of women do it, you know." Her statement provides a clear reflection of how she incorporated the communal identity of mother into her self-concept. However, in her postpartum experience, she quickly realized she could not work immediately after having her child. Mimi also talked about the expectations she had for herself, discussing how even though she was grieving the loss of her mother (who passed away while Mimi was pregnant), Mimi felt responsible for keeping her house clean, taking steps to get back to her pre-baby weight, and making sure she and her husband were in a positive relational space. She went on to say that despite her preparations and expectations for herself, she still experienced postpartum depression.

The communal identity of a postpartum mother is one where a woman delivers her child naturally and through vaginal birth, desires and succeeds in breastfeeding her infant, finds joy and fulfillment in mothering that makes up for the hardships, and can be successful at work and home. Interestingly, most of those I spoke with described pieces of this identity in relation to their own experience and how the two did not align. Indeed, mothers felt identity tensions in comparing themselves to other mothers.

Personal-Communal Gap: The Comparison Trap

Ellen always thought she would be a stay-at-home mom. Reflecting on her experience, she told me:

> The most devastating part of it all, and it still is devastating to think about it, and still coming to terms with it, is growing up I always thought career-wise, I was going to be a mom. Like I was gonna be a mom, and I'm going to stay at home with my kids, and I'm going to love it. Like my mom did. And I always said like if I could be half the mom my mom is. I mean my mom . . . she was like a baby whisperer, if you were to meet her. If I were half the mom that she was, I would feel accomplished. And I was not, that was just not happening.

I identified a gap between the personal and communal layers when women discussed their own experiences compared to the perceived experiences of others, which were filtered through a communal identity of a "mother." Often, these women referenced their expectations for motherhood, which were influenced by both their perceived experiences of others and ideologies about motherhood, compared to their actual lived experiences as mothers. In the quote above, Ellen invokes the personal, relational, and communal layers of identity. She first shares how she saw her self-identity once she became a mom. Then, she talks about how she perceived her own mother's identity in her role as a mother. However, there are clear communal identities present in Ellen's talk, reflecting the communal identity of "mother." Ellen sees her mother's identity as aligned with the communal identity of a mother, yet Ellen's own experience left her not feeling the self-worth she thought she would feel once she became a mother.

Similarly, Hannah talked about how her mother-in-law's perception of what a mother should be conflicted with Hannah's own identity. Unlike Ellen, she did not express a wish to have this identity; however, she still felt a conflict. She said:

> Uhm, my mother-in-law is definitely kind of that other side of just like I should have a perfectly clean house. Everyone should be dressed and ready to go by like 8:00 o'clock in the morning. I should have full makeup and full everything perfect. And dinner for everyone, every night, like home meat and potato meals. And if her son, my husband, is not getting that every night, then I'm not doing my job. So I do feel that pressure from her because she is someone who I value, you know, how she thinks about me, and how her son's getting treated.

Again, the relational identity present in communication from Hannah's mother-in-law was in alignment with a communal identity of mother; however, Hannah's self-concept was not in alignment with these two layers, creating what Hannah described as "pressure" from her mother-in-law to perform an identity she didn't associate with in order to maintain a positive relationship identity with her mother-in-law. Indeed, "by definition, the nontraditional personal identity will be at odds with the associated normative communal identity" (Maeda & Hecht, 2012, p. 48). Hannah's nontraditional personal identity as a mother, where she didn't feel a desire to be in charge of all home management, was at odds with the traditional communal identity of motherhood.

Mothers and mothers-in-law were not the only persons women compared themselves to. Women also discussed their friends and social circles and how these influenced their vision of themselves as mothers. Julia said:

> I would say because I run in musician and artist circles, there's lots of granola-crunchy moms that you know have their babies slung and whipping them out at festivals and stuff. So that's like what I saw, and I was like that's kind of like, "That's what I would like." I want him around and be able to experience these things and, you know, like I was envisioning a fantasy of the kind of mother I was going to be, I think, and trying to live that out.

Julia specifically discussed her struggles with breastfeeding and how she had envisioned herself as a mom who would breastfeed her children but then was not able to reach her breastfeeding goals. Again, Julia connects her self-concept as a mother to her friends but also invokes a communal identity of the "granola-crunchy mom," assuming that by using that phrase, I and others would be able to conjure an understanding of what a granola-crunchy mom is.

Furthermore, women discussed having expectations of motherhood that, when faced with their reality, did not align. Ellen said, "That is just devastating to have all those, you know thoughts and experiences when you go in with these expectations, of what motherhood is going to be like for you. And then it's just ppsshhhh." Ellen does not compare herself specifically to another mother but rather references a general communal identity of motherhood and the expectations she internalized as part of that. Bethany mentioned seeing pictures and stories of women breastfeeding and wanting to be able to breastfeed herself, but medical issues prevented her from reaching her breastfeeding goals. In all these instances, women compared their own experiences to those of "other women" or "other moms," drawing on a communal identity of motherhood.

Conclusion

"Mother" is a role we embody and an identity we may or may not associate with. Mother as a social identity has certain behavioral and communicative scripts that go along with that role, as articulated by the constructs of intensive mothering (Hays, 1996), competitive mothering (McHenry & Shultz, 2014), and combative mothering (Moore & Abetz, 2016). Indeed, the idea of motherhood is shaped not only by personal ideas and beliefs but also through social interactions and institutions (Alford, 2019). When one thinks of a "mother," certain cultural expectations inevitably come to mind. Once a woman internalizes the identity of "mother," she looks to the designated scripts assigned to that identity and incorporates them into her sense of self. Mothers also group themselves into ingroups and outgroups compared to other mothers along lines such as career status (Rittenour & Odenweller, 2019). Not only do mothers group themselves based on their mothering identity, but they also are grouped by others into the mother identity. For example, as a woman becomes a mother and returns to work, due to her new role identity, she may face stereotyping by others that she will prioritize family considerations over her career and, as a result, may be excluded from consideration for promotions or other opportunities.

In their talk, those I spoke with used terms such as "as a mother, you will . . ." to represent a communal identity of mother. Here, women described societal images of identity and how their identity changes when they become mothers. Importantly, unlike the other layers, the women I talked with mainly described the expectations they had going into motherhood and how those were not met by reality. As the communal layer represents an identity that is jointly remembered and taught to new members (Hecht, 2015), it makes sense that the expectations those I spoke with describe about motherhood, specifically when they discuss learning those expectations from society, would fall into the communal layer of identity.

The communal identity of ideal postpartum mothering materialized clearly through the discussions I had. The women participating in interviews with me communicated a communal identity of ideal postpartum mothering as: *mothers deliver their child without complications and heal quickly from childbirth*; *mothers feel a natural and instant connection with their infant*; *mothers want to breastfeed their children and do so without complications*; *mothers feel extreme joy in motherhood which makes up for the difficulty of mothering*; *being a mother becomes the most fulfilling role and priority for women*; and *mothers can manage taking care of their child(ren), running their house, and excelling in their careers*. Even as women experienced postpartum depression, this was the ideal of a postpartum mother that they incorporated into their understanding of how they would be a mother and experience mothering.

Broader cultural narratives and social messages reinforce this communal identity. For example, Rowe and Fisher (2015) found that pregnant women feel personally responsible for the outcome of their pregnancy. Scharp and Thomas (2017) identified a dominant discourse present in narratives of women with postpartum depression that mothers immediately fall in love and bond with their infant after birth. Regarding infant feeding, the most common message mothers receive is "breast is best" (Hosek et al., 2021). In their study on the performance of motherhood, DeGroot and Vik (2019) shared how mothers indicated that the conversations they had with others about parenting prior to becoming mothers had a positive spin. American ideologies of intensive mothering and ideologies about women's biological state reflect the idea that a woman will find the most fulfillment by birthing and caring for her child (Glenn, 1994; Hays, 1996). Hays (1996) also discussed the notion of supermom in her book on intensive mothering, where mothers have the option to stay at home full-time or work, but either way, they still must prioritize child-rearing. All these messages about what motherhood is like and how one should be as a mother that come from larger societal ideologies represent a commonly held view, or communal identity, of a mother.

However, these idealized expectations often stand in stark contrast to the lived realities of mothers. Those I spoke to described these expectations in light of how their lived reality fell short of their expectations. Indeed, while the traditional narrative of motherhood frames it as a time of excitement, affection, and positive change, "it is evident that this narrative is at best an embellishment and at worst a falsification of the reality many women face in early motherhood" (Elliott et al., 2020, p. 2). Certainly, the lived experience of mothers reveals a more complex and often difficult picture. The experiences of mothers reveal challenges such as breastfeeding difficulties, overwhelming responsibilities, emotional exhaustion, and the struggle to balance personal time with childcare, alongside the intense connection they feel with their children, which can be both a source of joy and stress (Constantinou et al., 2021). Mothers often make social comparisons, especially with other mothers, regarding their competence in managing the challenges to their careers and appearances that arise post-motherhood (Rittenour & Odenweller, 2019; Tosun et al., 2020). This struggle is exacerbated by the pervasive idealization of motherhood, where mothers are expected to be constantly available to their children while simultaneously maintaining professional success—a fundamentally contradictory expectation.

The consequences of this idealization are significant. When mothers don't live up to the ideals of intensive mothering, they feel they are not good enough (Cronin-Fisher & Parcell, 2019). Cronin-Fisher and Parcell (2019) found that mothers experience dissatisfaction as they transition to motherhood; however, they write that the ideology of intensive mothering (i.e., communal identity) likely keeps many women from sharing their dissatisfaction. Within intensive mothering, mothers are expected to feel joy and fulfillment in their role as mothers; dissatisfaction does not align with the accepted form of mothering communicated by the intensive mothering discourse.

These mismatches between communal identity and lived experience can affect maternal mental health. The pressure to meet societal expectations can significantly affect how women perceive their connection to their infants and their confidence in their mothering abilities (Fenwick et al., 2008). When mothers who have postpartum depression are unable to meet their idealized expectations of what motherhood is supposed to be like, they isolate themselves due to shame or guilt (Mollard, 2014). Furthermore, crushed maternal expectations are "an essential contributing factor to women developing postpartum depression" (Mollard, 2014, p. 661). Therefore, perhaps understanding the communal identity of a postpartum mother and the identity tensions between the communal identity and other layers is essential to our understanding of postpartum depression.

Chapter Summary

The communal layer of identity comprises cultural ideas and ideologies about identities, as well as the behavioral scripts that correspond to those identities. The women I spoke with in my research shared a clear and common understanding of what it meant to be a "good" postpartum mother. Through their conversations, they indicated how this concept was shaped by societal and interpersonal messages. Women were taught that an ideal postpartum mother delivers her child vaginally and without complications, has a natural and instant connection with her child, breastfeeds easily and willingly, will find true joy and fulfillment in mothering that will make up for any challenges, and can "do it all."

As mothers compared themselves to other mothers they knew or a generalized ideal of motherhood, they found themselves feeling like they didn't measure up. Within CTI, I identified this as a personal-communal gap. Women discussed identity tensions related to breastfeeding, staying at home full-time, and expectations from others, among other experiences. The communal identity of mother is shaped and reinforced, in part, through broad cultural narratives. However, the communal identity of mother often represents an idealized and unattainable version of motherhood. When women cannot live up to this idealized version, their expectations of what being a mother would be like are crushed. As crushed maternal expectations are a contributing factor to postpartum depression (Mollard, 2014), exposing ideologies related to the communal identity of mother can be valuable in understanding why and how women face those crushed expectations.

5

The Relational Self—Messages from Others, Our Relationships, and the Impacts on Mothering Identity amid Postpartum Depression

Eva's husband was supportive in both of her postpartum periods. She told me that when he had to return to work after one week of paternity leave, he "did everything he could" to find someone to stay at home with Eva for another week or two. He supported Eva as she struggled with postpartum depression, sleep deprivation, and breastfeeding struggles.

And yet, when I asked Eva if any events stood out in her mind that made her realize she had some sort of postpartum depression, she told me a story of how, one night, her newborn son would not sleep. Eva decided to put her son in the car and start driving, as this usually helped her baby calm down. After her son finally fell asleep, she pulled over. She told me what happened next, saying:

> I was in the parking lot of our, like our local park, and I remember emailing my husband this crazed—just all these thoughts about like wanting to get divorced and how I didn't feel like he was helping me, and how I was so tired, and you know, this wasn't what I thought it was going to be. And at that point, I think writing out how I was feeling—I didn't really intend to do it. It just happened—and I was also angry. I was angry that he could go to work, and I couldn't go to work and get away. And I think I was, I was jealous almost. And I think that's when I thought to myself, like, something is wrong.

Eva and her husband did not get divorced. In fact, she later told me their relationship was stronger than ever. I could relate to Eva's story. I told Eva that I had also experienced jealousy toward my husband. Like Eva, I was jealous that he could go to work, and I couldn't.

My own "aha" moment was when I was dealing with a colicky, crying baby. I put my son down in his crib, stomped into our bedroom, and screamed at my husband, "Why the FUCK aren't you helping me?!" (or something along those lines—I distinctly remember screaming the f-word at him; however, I can't remember if it was a question or a demand). My husband had no idea I needed help. It was my shift with our son, and the baby was simply crying. My husband didn't understand how triggering my son's cries were to me. Like Eva, I had feelings of tension in my relationship and distinctly remember thinking I was going to get divorced because who would want to be married to someone as miserable as me? These thoughts, though symptoms of postpartum depression, crept deep into my sense of self and my identity within my marriage.

Eva's story, my story, and the experiences of the other women I interviewed highlight the complex ways in which postpartum depression penetrates relationships and identities. In the relational layer of identity, "identity is a mutual product, jointly negotiated and mutually formed in relationships through communication" (Hecht et al., 2005, p. 263). The relational layer of identity has its foundations in symbolic interactionism and role theory (Hecht, 2015).

The relational layer of identity takes three forms. First, there is ascribed relational identity, which is internalizing how others view oneself (someone may tell you that you are an empathetic person, and you internalize that perception) (Jung & Hecht, 2004). Second, there is role identity, which is defined as one's identity relative to a relational role (Colaner et al., 2014) or one's identity in relation to a relational partner ("I am so-and-so's mother"). Finally, a relationship itself can be an identity, such as a couple or family unit (Hecht et al., 2005).

The relational layer of identity presented in ways that aligned with other layers of identity and in ways that presented identity gaps for participants. In *ascribed relational identity*, I focus on the identity-confirming messages received from other mothers. In *role identity*, I focus on how participants discussed to whom they disclosed their postpartum depression based on their relationship with that person. Finally, for *relationship identity*, I focus on the marital identity described by participants. Following these descriptions, I describe *identity gaps* related to the relational layer of identity.

Ascribed Relational Identity: Supportive Messages from Other Mothers

Cierra told me going to a postpartum depression support group was critical for her healing, saying, "Having other moms tell me this is exactly what I went through too, and it's normal, was like the biggest relief. It was like the biggest catharsis." Cierra's statement shows how she felt normal when others told her that her experience was common.

Part of relational identity is ascribed relational identity, which refers to the identity others ascribe to us. We form our sense of our ascribed identities based on our communication with others; how others interact with us conveys messages about how they perceive us. The mothers I spoke with talked about receiving supportive and/or validating messages from other mothers related to postpartum depression struggles that aligned with their own desired self-concept as a mother; namely, that they were not unusual in experiencing depressive symptoms, and it did not make them a bad mother.

For example, Katherine mentioned how when she disclosed her postpartum depression and anxiety on social media, she received positive feedback from others. "There were women, and I mean I knew them personally, but not close friends, not people that I had confided in or that messaged me texts, sent text messages. 'You know, if you ever need to talk, like I had it, I've been there, I fought through it all alone, there's no reason for you to fight through it alone.'"

Other mothers confirmed Katherine's postpartum depression experience when they shared that they also experienced postpartum depression, therefore helping her fit her own experience as a mother into other's experiences as mothers. In addition to support groups and friends, some of those I interviewed shared how their own mothers were helpful in the messages they shared. Hannah talked about how her mother confirmed her experience and identity, saying her mother told her, "I'm doing such a great job and . . . you have good days, and you have hard days. You have a lot of both. But just that I'm doing great." When mothers who are struggling hear messages like, "You're doing great," they may intake those messages within an ascribed identity.

When mothers received supportive messages from other mothers, these messages were identity-confirming in that they helped the participant make sense of their postpartum depression in relation to their identity as a mother. All but two[1] of the participants mentioned receiving supportive messages from other mothers. These messages came from their own mothers, other family members, friends, and support groups.

Relational Identity: Negotiating Disclosure

When asked about disclosing her postpartum depression to others, Cierra reflected how she told her husband but not her parents, saying, "I didn't really tell them any of the details, 'cause it's just not the way it is in my family." She connects her familial identity with her enacted identity. In this case, Cierra aligned her enacted identity with her relational familial identity by not discussing personal mental health issues with her family members.

Mothers reflecting on their experiences discussed disclosing (or not) their postpartum depression symptoms or diagnosis to their partner, their own mother or parents, grandmother, and friends. The choice to disclose was clearly connected to the person's various relationship identities and whether they felt able to enact an identity as someone experiencing postpartum depression symptoms to that relational partner.

Many of the women I spoke with mentioned a close relationship with their own mothers and had positive experiences when disclosing their postpartum depression symptoms to them. Ashley talked about how her relationship with her mother affected her choice to disclose, saying, "My mom and I are best friends. I'm always just very transparent with her." Ashley also described her

[1] The two women who did not mention receiving supportive messages from other mothers also said they did not disclose their postpartum depression to anyone.

mother as "very empathetic, very supportive" when Ashley was struggling with postpartum depression. By being empathetic and supportive, Ashley's mother was essentially communicating that experiencing postpartum depression was not diminishing Ashley's identity as a mother. When preparing to disclose a stigmatized invisible illness, there is a greater expectation of support based on the closeness between the two persons (Choi et al., 2016). Therefore, it makes sense that when individuals felt close to their mothers, they disclosed to them.

Additionally, the mothers I talked with shared how, after they disclosed their postpartum depression, their mothers provided tangible and emotional support. Lara's mother accompanied her to the doctor and served as her advocate during the appointment. Other women's mothers served as a sounding board, where women could ask their mothers questions or talk to them anytime about their experiences.

Mothers did not necessarily have to know the "right" supportive messages to say when their daughters disclosed their postpartum depression in order to be perceived as supportive. For example, Ellen mentioned how when she told her mother about her depression, rather than saying something, the fact that her mother did not say anything was helpful. Ellen said, "But she didn't respond with like a, 'You shouldn't feel that way. What's wrong with you?' Yeah, she really had no response, which I think was the perfect response." Maria talked about how even though her mother didn't always say or do support "right," she was still helpful, saying, "She listened to me. Even though she wouldn't always do it right, obviously. But she tried, and she was consistently there anytime I called, or she allowed me to just talk for forever annoyingly about the same stupid stuff that has happened." In these instances, the lack of judgment, the sharing of similar experiences, and empathetic responses were what mothers felt were supportive.

While within my interviews, this was more the exception than the rule, some women did not disclose their postpartum depression to anyone (at least, at first). In these cases, the women mentioned the stigma associated with postpartum depression. For example, Annisa said, "I didn't talk to anyone. Because you know, culturally, it's a terrible, terrible thing to talk about that." She connected the choice to disclose not only to the anticipated response from those close to her but also to the cultural norms in her home country surrounding mental health, which penetrates the communal layer of identity.

Dawn also linked her choice to not talk to anyone to the stigma associated with postpartum depression, saying,

> But with my oldest, I didn't talk to anybody about it cause I thought that it was—like I had heard of it before, but I didn't know too much about it. So I thought that the thoughts I was having were so far out there that somebody would take her from me, and that was like my biggest fear, so I didn't tell anybody for eight months.

At times, other women tried to hide their postpartum depression by not disclosing it to others. Grace said she did not tell her grandmother because "My Nana had a weird view of mental health. She was 90," again, connecting her choice to not disclose to the perceived receptiveness of the person she was disclosing to—illuminating how her relational identity and enacted identity interpenetrated in this decision.

Relationship Identity: Marital Relational Identity

Eva credits her struggle with postpartum depression as strengthening her romantic relationship with her husband. She told me, "I think it's actually made our marriage stronger, even though we did go through a period that was pretty hard." Other women spoke about how their partners validated their feelings, helped with childcare and household duties, and, like Eva, formed a stronger relationship with them.

While not all the women I spoke with identified as heterosexual, all had their child with their male romantic partner, and all but two were married to the father of their child(ren). Experiences within marital relational identity varied, sometimes within the same relationship. For analytical purposes, in the current section, I describe instances where marital identity positively aligned with other layers as women experienced postpartum depression. I then describe the gaps in the next section.

During the time they were experiencing postpartum depression, women mentioned how their partners supported them both emotionally and tangibly. The emotional support came in the form of supportive messages, such as when Ellen said, "He never once told me that I was overreacting or that there was something wrong with me or anything like that. Like he was there. He was in it, and he was very supportive of me." These types of supportive messages can be confirming for both the ascribed relational identity level and the relationship identity level.

In addition to emotional support, several mothers described how their postpartum depression necessitated that their partner take on more of the tangible duties of child and home care. For example, Bethany said:

> I think one of the things that has been really—that was really good I think in retrospect is because I couldn't really take care of my son very well in the beginning, I allowed him to do more maybe than if I would have been really competent at the beginning. So you know, I'm really thankful; I ask him to do things all the time and probably pre-child I really didn't do that you know? Because I just took care of it myself.

Bethany describes how experiencing postpartum depression necessitated better communication and delegation of duties between her and her husband, hence shaping their joint marital identity. Similarly, Ellen discussed how not only did her husband support her emotionally but also took on a large amount of child and home care when she was experiencing her depression in order for Ellen to focus on issues such as addressing her insomnia with healthcare professionals. By making these tangible changes in home responsibility, the marital identity changed. Indeed, Mimi described the changing dynamics of her marital relationship, saying, "He can kind of see that there are certain things that need to be done to take care of our son and so he preeminently does some things without me having to ask." Interestingly, the interviewees described these workload distribution changes in the marital relationship as lasting, not just something that happened while mothers were going through their postpartum depression.

Finally, some women talked about their postpartum depression experience as a shared struggle with their partner that led to a more positive understanding between the couple. In Eva's experience, her postpartum depression created tension within the relationship, but overcoming the challenge together ultimately strengthened their relationship. Dawn talked about how, prior to her postpartum depression, she and her husband may have argued with each other when one of them was going through an anxiety issue, whereas now, they understand each other's mental health. Similarly, other participants discussed how the experience strengthened their relationships as communication was enhanced and talking about feelings became normalized. Several participants specifically spoke about how their husband came from a family of origin where they "did not talk about feelings," and postpartum depression enabled the couple to normalize sharing feelings within their own relationship.

Despite the positive manifestations of relational identity during their experience with postpartum depression, the women I interviewed also experienced tensions between their relational identity and other layers of identity. They felt gaps in identity when their experiences were dismissed or downplayed by others when they felt resentment that their partner's life did not change as fundamentally as theirs', and when they felt their partner was expecting them to adhere to a stereotype of wife and mother to which they themselves did not ascribe.

Personal-Relational Gap: Negating of Mother's Postpartum Depression Identity

As she related her experience with postpartum depression, Mimi described feeling that her husband was frustrated with her, saying:

> He doesn't say it, and he's never said it, but I feel like that you know other people are able to do this. And I just feel like if I ask him to, you know, "Can you just hold the baby?" or whatever, like the look on his face or the, "Can I go to the bathroom first?" or "Can I take my shoes off?" or whatever. And I just want to say to him like, you know, "I don't get to do any of those things all day long through the day." I don't get to go to the bathroom by myself. I don't get to eat a sandwich by myself.

Whether or not Mimi's husband was actually frustrated, Mimi perceived that he felt like other mothers could do it all, and she could not. However, Mimi also shared how her husband was supportive of her during her postpartum and how their relationship had been strengthened due to their shared postpartum struggles. Indeed, mothers can experience support and tension within the same relationship as parents navigate the complicated task of infant care along with the added burden of postpartum depression.

Similar to Mimi's experience, the most common identity gap mentioned by the women I spoke with was the experience where they shared their symptoms, were truthful about their postpartum feelings, or attempted to receive treatment for their symptoms and were dismissed, or others negated their identities. I conceptualize this experience as an identity gap between the personal and relational layers of identity. Jung and Hecht (2008) define the personal-relational gap as the difference between an individual's self-view and their perception of how others view them. Mothers were sharing their personal experiences and postpartum struggles, i.e., how postpartum depression was felt within their selves. Then, this experience was negated by messages from others, where others dismissed mothers' postpartum depression symptoms or communicated that mothers were wrong in feeling the way they were feeling. Mothers were given messages such as they were not really experiencing postpartum depression; rather, they "had the Baby Blues," they were acting ungrateful, or they just needed sleep.

First, some women experienced a personal-relational gap when they told their husbands about their feelings, communicated a need for support, or suggested that they might have postpartum depression. Various women I talked to discussed how their husbands were not recognizing the support that they needed while they were communicating their postpartum depression. Ashley talked about her husband's views on depression, saying, "I'm not totally convinced that he even believes in depression or if what I'm feeling is, you know, normal." By not recognizing depression as real, Ashley's husband was not accepting her illness as an authentic experience.

Other mothers also felt unsupported by their husbands at times when they were struggling with postpartum depression symptoms. Lara told a specific story that she felt affected her relationship with her former husband, saying, "I remember calling [ex-husband] and I'm like, 'You've got to come home from work; like I'm losing my mind.' And . . . he was like, 'Just go tell my mom that you need help.' And I was like, 'I don't want to tell your mom that I need help; like I want you to come home.' He wouldn't." In these instances, mothers were facing struggles related to their postpartum depression, reaching out to their husbands for support, and not receiving the desired support from their husbands. This experience created an identity gap, where mothers felt that their personal experiences were not validated by their spouses and within their marital relationships. In some cases, women mentioned both support and non-support from their husbands, showing that the relationship and influence on identity fluctuated during their experience.

In addition to their marital partners, mothers also discussed messages from other family members, including their own mother, that impacted their experience. Most women discussed their experiences with their mothers as positive and aligned with their identity layers. However, some recollected experiences with their own mothers that manifested as identity gaps. Eva recollected how her mother was unsupportive when she disclosed that she was experiencing depressive symptoms, saying, "Her responses were very cold. They were very, you know, 'When you become a mother, this is what you signed up for, and it's going to be a lifetime of worrying and it's going to be a lifetime of, you know, anxiety.'"

The response to Eva's experience is particularly interesting because her mother frames her struggles not as postpartum depression but simply as part of motherhood, which, as her mother states, is "what she signed up for." Eva went on to discuss how she sought out more supportive messages from other relational partners, including her husband. Similarly, other women mentioned that their mothers did not express emotional support or implied that they were being ungrateful.

Finally, the mothers I spoke with discussed how their symptoms were negated or framed as outliers by medical professionals. This is particularly concerning, considering health professionals treat women with postpartum depression. Maria talked about how it took her several tries to find a therapist whom she trusted. Furthermore, Maria mentioned not being able to trust other healthcare providers, saying, "And being Black and having a white doctor, I didn't feel there was a real like connection between the two of us based on some of our conversations." Maria calls on her personal identity as a Black woman related to her relationship with her OBGYN to explain the tension.

Dawn also discussed the difficulty of not being able to trust doctors during the prenatal process. She faced a traumatic experience when she went to the emergency room while pregnant, and the emergency room doctor dismissed her thoughts on her condition. Even before she experienced postpartum depression, her previous experience with healthcare professionals led to an identity tension where medical providers invalidated her experience.

Other mothers in this study also reported not receiving the care they desired from healthcare providers. Hannah reflected on her gender identity impacting her interaction with medical providers, saying, "Like this sounds bad, but I feel like there's just again, like, a society view of women just being more dramatic when they're pregnant. Like, oh, it's just hormones, and you know, and like it's taken less seriously sometimes because it's like women are just being overboard with emotion." Here, she reflects on a societal attitude about women and emotions. Relationships with healthcare providers can be influenced by women's salient social identities, including gender and race.

Isabella shared that her doctors were not helpful in treating her postpartum depression when the basic treatment methods (medicine and therapy) did not help. Bethany also discussed how when she sought treatment, she felt like there wasn't a good treatment option for mothers experiencing postpartum depression. While not all mothers in the study experienced a lack of desired care and treatment by healthcare professionals, when they did, it only created more identity problems for them as a mother who felt she was experiencing postpartum depression to be dismissed as "untreatable" or be told that she was not having postpartum depression symptoms.

Relational-Relational and Relational-Communal: Gaps Related to the Spousal Relationship Identity

Several days after the birth of their child, Annisa's husband went abroad to continue his education, something Annisa and her husband had initially planned to do together. Instead, Annisa stayed in their home country to care for their child. Eventually, she joined her husband, but during her time postpartum, she felt envious that her husband was able to continue to do the things he had planned to do, while her life completely changed after having their child. She said, "I always thought at that time, like, not fair, you know? Like I was very envious to my husband, like you know, he gets to continue his education, he can have friends, you know, he can go outside. I went outside but a different way, right? We had a stroller."

Annisa was just one of several women I spoke with who reflected on feeling resentful that their husbands could work outside the home. Other women shared similar feelings, mentioning that they felt angry or jealous because their husbands could work outside the home, while they felt limited to staying at home. These women all had jobs or were students outside the home, and after the birth of their child, they took maternity leave or stayed at home with their child. Through this talk, I identified evidence of a gap within the relational layer of identity. Women felt a loss of their previous roles as they took on the role of mother, while at the same time, they saw that their husbands did not experience this loss. This led them to disconnect from their husband through negative feelings such as resentment or jealousy. I conceptualize these tensions as a relational-relational gap because of how mothers experienced their role as mothers and how it fits into their marital relationship, along with their husband's role as fathers.

Another gap related to the spousal relational identity was evident in how gender roles manifested within the postpartum experience. Sometimes, women connected this to the fact that their husbands were returning to work and, therefore, not participating in infant care. For example, Isabella mentioned feeling resentful that her husband could go to work and was not participating in the difficult parts of infant care. She described her feelings as, "Uhm, kind of like resentment, especially towards my husband who was able to work outside the home. And could, you know, either could not or like would not take on some of the like, nighttime feeding and stuff."

Similarly, Hannah mentioned feeling resentment toward her husband because he did not participate in the care of their infant, saying:

> I feel like he just didn't even know like what to do. And I didn't necessarily know what to do either. So it was like I'm trying to figure it out, and I don't have the ability to also teach you what you need to do. Like just do it. Like just do like whatever you're thinking about . . . Just you, just go ahead and do it. 'Cause it's like I don't know what I'm doing either. So that was really frustrating the first go round because he was just kind of like, "Well, I don't have a boob, so there's nothing for me to do."

Here, Hannah demonstrates how her husband assumed she would instinctively know what to do in caring for their infant, presumably because of her identity as a "mother." In contrast, it is not expected that a man should instinctively know what to do as a "father." She counters this by saying that she didn't know what she was doing either. Other women mentioned feeling resentful that they were left to bear the sole burden of caring for their infant. I conceptualize these experiences as a gap between the relational and communal layers of identity. Here, a gap is evident in how participants felt care and responsibility would happen based on their relational identity with their husbands; however, clear ideas about gender roles related to mothering and infant care came into play.

Conclusion

In this chapter, I discuss how identity manifested in the relational layer during postpartum depression. Specifically, I examined how mothers navigated ascribed relational identity, relational identity, and relationship identity. I also analyzed the identity gaps that emerged—between personal and relational layers, within the relational layer itself, and between relational and communal layers—to show how identity disruptions can compound during the postpartum period. Now, I will discuss the implications of these observations on identity layers and the understanding of postpartum depression through a communicative framework.

Ascribed Relational Identity

To begin, within the ascribed relational layer, women's maternal identity was confirmed/supported when they received supportive messages from other mothers about their postpartum depression, such as normalizing their experience or that postpartum depression did not make them bad mothers. When women mentioned receiving positive support from others, they used phrases such as "she never judged me" or discussed how hearing from other mothers who had similar experiences was helpful. Theoretically, it makes sense that receiving supportive messages from other mothers would be a positive manifestation of identity. Through hearing from other mothers who had been through similar experiences, women were able to see themselves as fitting in with the social group of "mother." Mothers "compare themselves to other mothers in their social networks" (Rittenour & Odenweller, 2019, p. 252) to situate themselves within their mothering identity.

When these women were met with positive comparison and lack of judgment, they were able to negotiate their identities as mothers while still experiencing identity-threatening challenges, such as postpartum depression. Indeed, mothers can feel safest disclosing their parental challenges to people they feel experienced similar challenges (Vik & DeGroot, 2021). These conclusions align with previous qualitative work on support and postpartum depression; in their synthesis study, Dennis and Chung-Lee (2006) found that the most desired treatment by mothers for postpartum depression was the opportunity to talk to someone who was an empathetic and nonjudgmental listener, and having support from other mothers and knowing they are not alone are important factors in recovering from postpartum depression.

Next, I discuss how women reflected on disclosing their postpartum depression and parental challenges to others based on the relationship they had with the target person and the perceived response they anticipated. This leads to the next piece of the relational layer: relational identity.

Relational Identity

For analytical purposes, I conceptualized disclosure decisions and conversations as part of relational identity. However, there are clear intersections into enacted identity. Here, I focus on the relational aspect of the disclosure decision and enactment. Depression and other mental health illnesses can be invisible identities. Therefore, an individual may choose to reveal or conceal this identity based on how they want to be perceived by others. Clearly, all the women with whom I spoke disclosed their postpartum depression to at least one person: me. Additionally, many of the women were involved in postpartum support groups. However, when reflecting on their experiences, the women varied in the ways they initially disclosed their anxiety, depression, and other symptoms to their family and friends. Individuals discussed disclosure of their postpartum depression in relation to the person(s) they were disclosing to and how they wanted to be perceived or understood by that person, their relationship identity with that person, and/or the anticipated response from the person.

Previous exploration into postpartum depression disclosure and treatment-seeking barriers identified identity reasons for not disclosing and/or seeking help, including negatively impacting family identity, shame, and stigma (Dennis & Chung-Lee, 2006). These identity reasons align with the experiences of the women I spoke with who talked about hiding their postpartum depression symptoms and/or diagnosis.

In mothers' choices to disclose or not disclose their identity as someone with postpartum depression, the enacted layer and the relational layer of identities were closely connected, showing how, while identity layers can be studied separately, in reality, they are always working in conjunction and interpenetrating (Hecht, 2005). The enacted layer of identity is informed through Goffman's work on dramaturgy and facework (Hecht, 2015), where when we communicate, we enact our identities. Goffman argued that how we perform (or enact) depends on the audience and that the audience and actor engage in a mutual performance. Therefore, it makes sense that disclosure decisions would manifest differently depending on the relational situation. More than just a general front-stage or back-stage self, the women were considering a relationship-specific self (McBride, 2018). Women disclosed to their family members when they felt their family members would be supportive or that the relationship norm was to talk about mental health. They did not disclose when they perceived their family members would exhibit judgment or other non-supportive responses.

Relationship Identity

I also looked at how relationship identity manifested in marital relationships as women were experiencing postpartum depression. As one of the tensions in different-sex marital relationships is inequity in household management and family work (DeGroot & Vik, 2020), it makes sense that mothers whose husbands took on more family care duties during this time felt an enhanced relationship identity. These positive impacts on relationships were lasting. By sharing their struggles and receiving support from their partners and/or mothers, the relationship was transformed. While these relationships may have experienced tension and strain as participants experienced postpartum depression, many mothers felt that they were able to form stronger bonds with their loved ones as a result of their experience. Indeed, couples who view each other as a team when it comes to stressful life events are more likely to support each other and invest in the relationship during hard times (Afifi & Harrison, 2018).

Personal-Relational Gap

The personal-relational identity gap women experienced aligns with previous research on postpartum depression, showing that partners, family members, and even healthcare professionals are reluctant to acknowledge and respond to a mother's emotional needs (Dennis & Chung-Lee, 2006). Interestingly, a discrepancy between our self-view and other's views of us and failure to receive positive reassurance from others are both associated with depression (Jung & Hecht, 2008). In these experiences, mothers experienced a discrepancy between their self-view (thinking they were experiencing anxiety and depression) and other's views (dismissing symptoms as something else). These observations align with previous research exploring identity gaps, where researchers identified a personal-relational identity gap when others denied a person's illness (Voorhees, 2022).

Previous research also points to the fact that family members lack an understanding of postpartum depression (Dennis & Chung-Lee, 2006). Henshaw et al. (2016) identified that fathers whose partners were high on depression scores felt they lacked the knowledge, support, resources, and skills to be supporters of their partner during postpartum depression. However, Vik and DeGroot (2021) found that mothers experiencing postpartum depression want emotional and tangible support from their partners. Furthermore, "relationship satisfaction hinges on receiving positive support" (Vik & DeGroot, 2021, p. 17). Based on previous research and some experiences discussed here, there is a disconnect between the desired support of mothers and how fathers feel they can support mothers, as well as fathers' understanding of postpartum depression. This disconnect can manifest in identity gaps for the mothers, as their personal experiences are not validated with support by their husbands. Additionally, as fathers whose partners have postpartum depression are more at risk of experiencing postpartum depression themselves (Eddy et al., 2019), the fact that fathers lack an understanding of the condition and how to support those who have it presents an alarming problem for the mental health of fathers, too.

Furthermore, in their study on postpartum depression and treatment barriers, Dennis and Chung-Lee (2006) found that one help-seeking barrier was that mothers assumed that their struggles were a normal part of motherhood. In the current context, messages from others sometimes reinforced this mental mindset, including one's own mother (such as Eva's mother's response). Additionally, dominant cultural discourses dictate that mothers should only have positive emotions about motherhood (Scharp & Thomas, 2017) and that mothers should not complain when they are dissatisfied (Cronin-Fisher & Parcell, 2019). The responses from these women's mothers came from their own ideas about mothering, passed down through cultural norms and ideals and within their own social circles.

Women also received disconfirming identity messages from healthcare providers. The experience with healthcare providers is complex; mothers interact on an interpersonal level with doctors, therapists, nurses, and other healthcare providers. However, the recollections shared with me indicated that strong intergroup dynamics were at play. For example, both Dawn and Maria connected their experience to their social identities as Black women. The CDC (2021) has identified racism as a serious threat to the health of minority populations, and structural racism is a root cause of racial health inequalities

(Bailey et al., 2017). In their study on the lived experiences of Black mothers who had a life-threatening health complication following the birth of their child, Canty (2022) reported mothers felt a lack of personal connection with their healthcare providers, did not receive the support or guidance they needed, and even referenced feeling like their condition was minimized. These findings align with the experiences of Black mothers in the current study when they sought healthcare for various complications and concerns.

Along with racism, gender bias is a problem in healthcare, where women's symptoms are downplayed and treated differently than when presented by a man (Pagan, 2018). The downplaying of symptoms by medical professionals can impact a woman's decision to seek treatment. Indeed, in their review of qualitative studies, Dennis and Chung-Lee (2006) write that "Not surprisingly, when health professionals minimized a mother's feelings and symptoms, she became reluctant to pursue treatment" (p. 326).

Spousal Relational Gaps

I identified additional identity gaps within women's experiences as they discussed their relationships with their spouses. Women discussed feeling resentment toward their husbands for the lack of perceived change in their husband's life and a lack of support from their husbands in caring for their infants. I conceptualized these as relational-relational and relational-communal identity gaps due to how the women referenced their new roles, their marital relationships, and the influences of communal identities, such as wife, mother, father, and husband, that infiltrated their individual experiences.

Vik and Hafting (2012) found that mothers with postpartum depression in their study felt a loss of self as they became mothers, related in part to missing their professional lives. In the current context, not only did women discuss missing their professional lives, but they compared their new life to the losses faced in their husband's life, where losses were perceived as little or none at all. Colaner et al. (2014), who first identified identity gaps within the relational-relational layer, argue that any time levels of the relational layer conflict with each other, there is a potential for a relational-relational gap.

My observations and analysis presented here support this argument, as when tension existed between relational levels, women experienced an identity gap.

Martial identity was threatened when participants felt resentment toward their husband for his ability to work outside the home and when gender ideologies about the care of infants infiltrated the relationship where mothers felt the husband should participate more in childcare, but the husband did not or could not. Whether husbands chose not to engage in childcare or whether structural constraints prevented them from participating (for example, it is not common for men in the United States to be able to take paternity leave and, therefore, must return to work only days after their child is born), communal ideologies about gender norms influenced gaps present here. Motherhood is expected to come naturally to women (Cronin-Fisher & Parcell, 2019). However, accounts from women in the current study support the idea that motherhood is learned, not natural (Cronin-Fisher & Parcell, 2019), and in alignment with similar research on experiences of postpartum depression (Vik & Hafting, 2012), some mothers felt a lack of support from their partner. Identifying these relational-relational and relational-communal identity gaps is important because identity gaps put people at risk of decreased relational satisfaction (Faulkner & Hecht, 2011), and identity gap experiences can be damaging to married couples' feelings about their relationship (Kennedy-Lightsey et al., 2015).

To conclude, the women I spoke with revealed how their identities as mothers, partners, and individuals were continuously shaped and sometimes strained through interactions with spouses, family members, peers, and healthcare providers. These findings reaffirm the importance of understanding postpartum depression not just as an individual health issue but as a relational, cultural, and communicative phenomenon.

Chapter Summary

The relational layer of identity is conceptualized in three levels: ascribed identity, relational (role) identity, and relationship identity. Within the cribed relational level, participants' maternal identity was confirmed/

supported when they received supportive messages from other mothers about their postpartum depression, such as what they were experiencing was normal and not something to be ashamed of or that postpartum depression did not make them a bad mother. Within the relational level, participants considered the perceived responses from relational others in their choices to disclose or not disclose their postpartum depression symptoms and diagnosis. Their relational role to the target partner and how they conceptualized the dynamics of their relationship were key in their disclosure decisions. Finally, within the relationship identity level, participants discussed ways that their postpartum depression strengthened their marital relationship, whether it was through better communication or more emotional and tangible support from their husbands. Identity gaps manifested between the personal and relational layers as women shared their experiences and symptoms and were dismissed, and within the relational layer as, they navigated parenting and support with their spouses.

6

Advancing Our Understanding of Identity as Communicative

One of my goals in conducting this research was to advance the understanding of identity as a communicative phenomenon. The current exploration into identity manifestations has several implications for the Communication Theory of Identity. First, I discuss how my work enhances understanding of the Relational and Communal Layers of Identity. Then, I discuss how the current work adds to the research on identity gaps.

Relational Layer of Identity

While the personal and enacted layers of identity are relatively standard in description, understanding, and study throughout CTI research, the relational and communal layers are not as clear. My work contributes to CTI by expanding our understanding of these layers and their integral role in identity. I begin by discussing how my work contributes to the scholarly understanding of the relational layer of identity.

The relational layer may be the most complicated identity frame within CTI due to the various theoretical levels within the relational layer. While most references to the relational layer discuss three levels, there are diverging descriptions of what comprises the relational layer. In Hecht's (1993) original conceptualization of CTI, he writes that "Identity is mutually constructed in social interaction. In this construction, identity emerges in relationships and becomes a property of the relationship because it is jointly negotiated" (p. 79). He goes on to frame the three levels of relational identity: how people define themselves in terms of *others* (e.g., "they say I am smart"), how people define themselves in terms of *relationships with others* (e.g., husband, wife, sister), and finally, *relationships themselves as identity* (e.g., romantic couple).

Later, Jung and Hecht (2004) describe four layers of relational identity: ascribed relational identity, role identity, identities as they exist in relation to one another, and relationships as identities. Kam and Hecht (2009) divide the relational frame of identity into two levels, describing the relational layer as "a multidimensional construct consisting of identities derived from membership in a relationship [(e.g., a marriage)] which may be called relationship identities, and those derived from ascriptions, which may be referred to as ascribed relational identity" (p. 474) (e.g., how someone else describes you). In other words, they distinguish between identities as formed *within relationships* from identities *ascribed by others.* These various definitions point to a lack of consensus on how the relational layer of identity is defined in CTI.

The relational identity layer is complex, but CTI theorists agree upon one thing: "A relational identity is formed in communication with others" (Jung, 2011, p. 317). However, as defined in CTI, all aspects of identity are formed in communication with others, as communication constitutes identity and vice versa in CTI. A key feature of CTI is that it focuses on how identity is processed through interaction (Hecht et al., 2005). Therefore, all identity layers involve communication with others, from the personal layer to the communal layer. The relational layer of identity needs to have a more specific focus than simply being an identity formed in communication with others. The relational layer could benefit from a more precise conceptualization that researchers could use moving forward. I propose a standard conceptualization of the relational layer of identity that can help researchers using CTI to understand better how identity manifests within different relational levels of identity and where identity tensions exist.

Based on previous research and my observations and evaluations in this book, I see a benefit to separating the relational layer of identity into two layers: *ascribed relational identity* and *relational identity* (see Table 1). While both constructs have been identified in previous CTI work (Kam & Hecht, 2009), there has been no consistent adoption of the understanding of the levels within the relational layer. In the following paragraphs, I define

Table 1 Communication Theory of Identity Layers, Redefined

Layer	Description
Personal	Self-concept, how we see ourselves
Enacted	Performance of identity
Ascribed relational	The messages we receive from others and how we interpret them as part of our identity
Relational	How individuals identify themselves by their relationships and relationships as identity units
Communal	Cultural ideals, how society defines an identity

ascribed relational identity and relational identity, share examples from my research, and describe the benefit of separating the relational layer in this way as a codified and agreed-upon approach to using CTI's identity layers for researchers going forward.

Ascribed Relational Identity

Ascribed relational identity is defined as one's identity as ascribed by others or how others see us (Jung & Hecht, 2004; Kam & Hecht, 2009). These messages can be direct: "You are a good mom," or more indirect: "You handled your child's temper tantrum really well." Both messages convey an ascribed identity of "good mother," implying that the person sending the message perceives the recipient as a good mother. In other words, ascribed relational identity has everything to do with the messages we receive from others and how we interpret them as part of our identity.

For example, in my research, mothers discussed receiving supportive messages from other mothers. While clear interpenetrations exist between ascribed relational and relational identities, I will first discuss the aspect of ascribed relational identity. These messages came from close relational partners, such as mothers of the mother, and more distant others, such as members of an online or in-person support group. These messages manifested in ascribed identity, such as when Hannah's mother told her that she was doing a good job as a mother. Additionally, in some cases, mothers mentioned that a lack of messages was beneficial to their identity, as when they did not receive judgment from others.

Another example of ascribed identity was evident in the personal-relational gap, where mothers expressed postpartum depression symptoms to another, whether that was a close relational partner or a healthcare provider, and the response they received was a different perceived explanation of what was happening to them. For example, when Eva disclosed her postpartum depression symptoms to her mother, she received the response that she was not experiencing postpartum depression; she was just unable to handle the maternal load (an ascribed identity). Multiple women mentioned their husbands perceiving them as a mother who couldn't do the tasks associated with motherhood rather than as someone going through depression.

An important aspect of ascribed relational identity is that we may receive communication about ourselves from anyone, not just those with whom we have established interpersonal relationships. Bergquist et al. (2019) identified that refugees experienced ascribed identity interactions within their host culture, in both positive messages and negative stereotyping from others. These messages were sometimes from strangers or more distant acquaintances, such as coworkers, rather than close relational partners, and yet they still impacted refugees' identity manifestations. The women I spoke with mentioned messages that stuck with them from lactation consultants, nurses, and online support groups, among others, indicating that a message does not have to be from a close relational partner for it to be retained within ascribed identity. The messages received from others retained in ascribed identity are often memorable messages or messages that prescribe rules of conduct or moral codes and are personally salient (Knapp et al., 1981). Indeed, positive or negative messages about motherhood can impact mothering identity (Hosek et al., 2021). While initially framed as positive, scholars have recently framed memorable messages as having both positive and negative impacts (Rubinsky & Cooke-Jackson, 2017). However, one also receives memorable messages from close relational partners, which points to the complex interpenetration of identity frames and how, in reality, the identity frames are continually operating together, if not necessarily in alignment.

Relational Identity

By separating ascribed relational identity from relational identity, relational identity can now be thought of as involving our close interpersonal relationships. The relational layer of identity involves how individuals identify themselves by their relationships (Kam & Hecht, 2009; Maeda & Hecht, 2012) such as mother, child, best friend, coworker, *and* relationships as identity units (for example, the statement "we are a loud family" draws on the family as a shared identity unit). This clarification also helps capture what some scholars have categorized as part of the communal layer. When relational identity considers our relationships with others, that can be in a group or a dyad. For example, family identity, couple identity, team identity, and support group identity can all be part of relational identity, allowing the focus on the communal layer to attend to larger societal conceptualizations of identities. Additionally, by separating relational identity from ascribed relational identity, scholars can investigate interpersonal relationships as part of identity, separate from messages from others, and how the two align or conflict.

Again, through my discussions, I identified examples of relational identity. Mothers choose whom to disclose or not disclose to based on their relational identity with that person. Additionally, mothers drew upon their marital relationship identity both when that identity aligned with other layers and in identity gaps, such as the relational-relational gap, where mothers experienced a gap within the relational layer as they made sense of their role as a postpartum mother in relation to their role as a wife, partner, and their husband's role as a father and partner. Mothers also experienced a personal-relational gap when they did not feel an instant bonding with their infant.

An example of an ascribed relational-relational identity gap would be when a person receives a message from a close relational partner that does not align with their relationship identity with that person. For example, while I labeled the experience of telling one's husband about postpartum depression symptoms and being dismissed as a personal-relational gap, there also is a strong chance the marital relational identity was salient within the experience, along with ascribed relational identity.

By focusing on the relational layer of identity in examining the identity gaps women experience with postpartum depression, I contribute to our understanding of the relational layer and how it can be separated into two distinct layers: ascribed relational identity and relational identity. Ascribed relational identity attends to the messages received from others and their impact on identity. Relational identity attends to how we situate ourselves in our relationships with others and relationship units as identities. Therefore, the relational layer would no longer have various levels, which, in the current explication of CTI, is the only layer to have levels. By examining the ascribed relational and relational identity frames separately, scholars can better identify tensions among these and other identity layers, thereby furthering our understanding of identity as a whole and how communication contributes to identity. Next, I discuss the implications of my work for our understanding of the communal layer of identity.

Communal Layer of Identity

The communal layer of identity remains a relatively underexamined layer in CTI research. This is, in part, due to how the layer is conceptualized and measured, as well as how CTI studies often focus on individual experiences rather than collective ones. The communal layer represents how society defines an identity, and we can learn about how society defines an identity through media representations, organizational studies, social media, and other means (Hecht, 2015). Indeed, Kam and Hecht (2009) write that communal identity "does not reflect individual perceptions of identities such as group memberships" (p. 458). Therefore, the communal identity is not the social identities that are salient to oneself but rather how society defines an identity. This book adds to CTI in that it provides (a) a useful way for scholars to explore the communal layer and (b) an understanding of how communal identity is shared within relationships and among society.

Through my work, I offer two ways to explore communal identity in studies using interviews with individuals (or dyads). First, scholars can examine the communal by looking closely at the study participants' discourse and identifying phrases that point to larger societal ideals. The women I interviewed used phrases such as "society tells us" and "we're all expected" when they discussed communal identity of a postpartum mother. Furthermore, communal identity was communicated to mothers by others, reflecting the idea that a communal identity is jointly held and taught to new members (Hecht, 1993). To illustrate, Ashley said, "I was always told . . ." when discussing the ideals of becoming a new mother.

For future scholars interested in studying the communal layer, language such as "it's natural," "society tells us," or "everyone knows" is a good indicator of communal identity at play. For example, in their research on mother/daughter dyads and breast cancer, Fisher and Wolf (2019) found that ideas about women as the carer of the family are "rhetorically naturalized and rendered invisible" (p. 269). Ascriptions, traits, and ideas about an identity described as natural or as passed down through society can be considered as part of the communal layer of identity in that they help us understand not only how the individual in question thinks of an identity but also how the larger community/society as whole thinks of an identity.

Second, incorporating social media into my discussions allowed me to understand the communal layer of identity. Rather than selecting posts to share with the people I interviewed or conducting an analysis of social media posts, I asked women to share social media posts with me through a survey. Then, I discussed the posts as part of the interview process. Through this, I was able to understand what these women were seeing on social media and how they incorporated these posts as part of their understanding of mothering and postpartum depression. What I found was that women either shared posts they liked or posts that they disagreed with and offered explanations for their thoughts based on their lived experience as mothers who had postpartum depression. By incorporating social media discussions into my interviews and examining discourses in my findings, I was able to identify how the communal layer of identity manifested, in part, for the women I spoke with. Specifically, I identified a communal identity of a postpartum mother circulating through ideas from others and social media posts. In all, my work supports a conceptualization of the communal layer of identity as the identity that society attributes to a social group or identity. My additions add direction for researchers to investigate and interpret the communal layer of identity in future CTI studies.

Furthermore, my conclusions contribute to the work on the communal layer by demonstrating how the communal layer of identity affects not only the individual but also relationships. Communal identities do not have to be held solely by those who identify as members within that group, which is an extension of the current conceptualization of this layer in most empirical work using CTI. Outside members can also hold communal identities about a particular group—we all have an idea of what it means to be a mother, even if we are not mothers ourselves. For example, some of those I interviewed perceived that their husband held the same ideas about a postpartum mother as they did. Hannah reflected on how her husband perceived her as knowing how to care for their infant because of her identity as a mother, indicating that the communal identity of postpartum mother not only resided in Hannah's mind but was also relevant to her husband and their marital relationship. Therefore, the communal identity of postpartum mothers interpenetrated not only the personal and enacted layers but also the relational layer. This was important because it helped me to identify gender norms circulating in relationships.

Additionally, women projected the communal identity of a mother onto other mothers, regardless of whether those mothers identified with it themselves. For example, Ellen saw her mother as representing an ideal of motherhood but didn't mention whether this was how her mother felt about herself. This is an example of how intensive mothering ideologies are reified through generations. Previous CTI studies have suggested that there are both individual and communal levels of all the identity layers (Hecht, 2015); my work here supports the notion that the communal layer of identity, or at least communal ideologies of an identity, interpenetrates all the layers.

The communal layer represents cultural ideals. While the personal layer encompasses the social identities one associates oneself with (Hecht, 2015), the communal layer shares a common overall social identity (Greenaway et al., 2018). Therefore, I argue, for example, that a soccer team's group identity is not a communal identity but a relational identity. Furthermore, family identity should fall under relational identity rather than communal identity. A communal identity is a general societal understanding of what a soccer player or a soccer team is (for example, "soccer players are athletic, confident, and good-looking" could represent a communal identity).

Stereotypes may especially come into play within the communal layer. For example, the stereotype of mothers with postpartum depression as not loving their children could be held not only by individuals with postpartum depression but also by their family members, friends, or even healthcare providers. By examining the communal layer as a cultural representation, we can understand not only how members within the group create, refine, and reference a communal identity but also how outside members cite communal identities in their interactions. Next, I consider how this text contributes to addressing identity gaps and promoting well-being.

Identity Gaps and Implications for Well-Being

Identity gaps are an aspect of interpenetration of identity layers and help us understand how various identity frames work together to form a dynamic identity (Jung & Hecht, 2004). Furthermore, identity gaps are described as an inevitable result of communication (Jung & Hecht, 2004) and have been associated with negative outcomes, including depression (Jung & Hecht, 2008), feeling misunderstood (Jung & Hecht, 2004), and decreased communication satisfaction (Jung, 2011; Jung & Hecht, 2004). However, identity gaps also can initiate positive identity change (Colaner et al., 2014; Hecht, 2015; Maeda & Hecht, 2012).

Considering identity gaps within the postpartum depression context is essential because "identity gaps formed in communication put people at risk for experiencing elevated levels of depression" (Jung & Hecht, 2008, p. 322). Indeed, in their study on identity gaps and depression among Korean immigrants, Jung and Hecht (2008) found that personal-enacted and personal-relational identity gaps are contributing factors to levels of depression. Furthermore, they identified the personal-relational identity gap as mediating situational factors on depression (Jung & Hecht, 2008).

While I did not aim to make predictions or generalizations about identity gaps and postpartum depression, the current text extends the work on identity gaps and well-being, providing direction for future research. First, I extended the examination of identity gaps and depression into the context of postpartum depression. To my knowledge, this is the first study of postpartum depression using CTI and identity gaps as a sensitizing theory. This is noteworthy because previous CTI research on identity gaps and depression shows that identity gaps are a significant explanatory construct for levels of depression (Jung et al., 2007). Therefore, there is a possibility that identity gaps and postpartum depression levels could be connected.

I identified not only what types of gaps may be forming within postpartum depression but also how those gaps manifest. For example, a personal-relational gap manifested when women shared their postpartum depression symptoms and received unconfirming identity messages in response and when women did not feel an identification with the role of mother. This is important because differences in how identity gaps are formed result in differences in the relationships between gaps and other variables (Jung & Hecht, 2008). Additionally, while researchers previously found that the enacted-relational and personal-relational gaps are not significant predictors of communication outcomes (Kam & Hecht, 2009), in the current context, the relational aspect of identity was an important part of mothers' experiences. Therefore, the salience of gaps related to the relational layer of identity may depend on the relational partner. For the women I interviewed, their husbands and mothers were significant relationships. Gaps developed within those relational identities may be more salient to experiences of depression or other adverse outcomes than gaps developed within relational identities of not-as-meaningful relationships.

Furthermore, Jung and Hecht (2008) found that identity gaps are a mediating function between situational stimuli and depression. This means that the situational stimuli were not a direct cause of levels of depression, but the stimuli contributed to the identity gap, which contributed to levels of depression. By exploring how identity gaps are formed during the postpartum depression experience, I provided insight into the societal and relational processes that may be contributing to that identity gap, which may offer insights into how the situational stimuli lead to an identity gap.

Finally, my work supports the notion that while identity gaps are associated with negative outcomes, they have the potential to initiate positive identity change (as posited by Colaner et al., 2014). Because I interviewed both women who were currently experiencing postpartum depression and women who had experienced postpartum depression in the past, I was able to explore the lasting effects of postpartum depression on identity. While there were some lasting effects that interviewees gave a negative valence to, such as continued mental health struggles and the decision not to have any more children, overall, the women I spoke with felt a positive impact on themselves and their relationships. In their study of always-single Japanese women over time, Maeda and Hecht (2012) identified that over time, as women negotiated identity gaps, the gaps were no longer necessarily negative. Indeed, women coped better with identity gaps over the years (Maeda & Hecht, 2012). In the current context, identity gaps may be threatening as women experience postpartum depression. However, gaps such as the personal-relational or relational-relational may require communicative work between relational partners for women to manage those tensions. That communicative work could, over time, lead to more positive relational outcomes, such as when Katherine said she and her husband understand each other's mental health as a result of her experience with postpartum depression.

In all, my work adds to the Communication Theory of Identity by (a) extending CTI into the context of postpartum depression, (b) showing the value of separating the relational layer of identity into ascribed relational and relational layers, (c) adding to understanding of how to conceptualize and study the communal layer of identity, and (d) providing valuable information on how identity gaps manifest during postpartum depression, which can guide researchers who want to explore postpartum depression and identity in future studies. In the next chapter, I discuss the implications of this work for research on postpartum depression and mothering.

Chapter Summary

I argue that the relational layer of identity, as conceptualized in CTI, should be separated into two layers: the ascribed relational layer of identity and the relational layer of identity. Ascribed relational identity should be thought of as one's identity as ascribed by others or how others see us. These messages can come from close relational partners. However, messages from acquaintances or even strangers may sometimes penetrate this layer, depending on the context. The relational layer of identity is the layer of identity that involves our close personal relationships. It includes both how individuals identify themselves by their relationships and relationships as identity units.

I suggest that the communal layer of identity can be examined by looking closely at discourse and identifying phrases that point to larger societal ideals, such as "it's natural," and through popular social media posts. As previously argued in CTI, the communal layer of identity expands beyond the individual. My research showed this in how the communal layer infiltrated relationships and how expectations of mothering identity were held in more than just the mother herself.

Through examining identity gaps, I was able to look at what types of identity gaps may be forming within postpartum depression and how those gaps manifest. Previous researchers have found that identity gaps have the potential to initiate positive identity change. My findings support this claim, as women reported positive long-lasting identity impacts of their experience with postpartum depression.

7

Where Do We Go from Here? Practical Implications for Healthcare Providers, Scholars, Family Members, and Mothers

Communication studies is a practical discipline—through research, scholars can improve communication practices as well as develop theory (Craig, 2018). By delving into the experiences of women affected by postpartum depression, I hoped to connect the theoretical concept of identity and identity gaps to practical advice and recommendations. Indeed, the experiences described and analyzed in this book offer valuable insights beyond just theory. In this chapter, I provide practical recommendations for healthcare providers, support persons, and mothers.

First, I suggest ways in which healthcare providers and others can talk to women about pregnancy, postpartum depression, and mothering. The way society and individuals communicate can significantly impact women's experiences and well-being, as I've shown through the testimonies included in the previous chapters. Second, I point to certain support persons as primary in the postpartum experience for the women I interviewed, namely, their romantic partners and their mothers. Understanding who plays a central support role in the postpartum period can help doctors, educators, friends, and family members better support new mothers. Finally, I offer practical implications for mothers as they situate themselves within their mothering identity. An identity shift is an important aspect of the transition to parenthood that deserves more attention.

Practical Application for Healthcare Providers: Take an Inclusive Approach to Discussions of Pregnancy and Mothering

When I was a new mom, a pediatrician told me to sleep-train my baby by letting her "cry it out" in between incrementally longer periods of time. However, I found this method unbearable—my daughter cried for hours, for nights on end, until my husband and I gave up this method of sleep training. With my son, I had the additional burden of postpartum depression/anxiety to deal with while listening to him cry. The sound of my son's cries was deeply triggering to me. Yet, no one gave me advice on how to handle that or even acknowledged the effect a baby's cries can have on a parent, despite research in biological brain imaging showing that the sound of one's baby crying triggers stress and anxiety responses in the brain (Swain et al., 2011). In much advice given to new mothers, whether it relates to safe sleep, delivery plans, or baby schedules, the parental experience often is not considered. But parents are not robots.

Mothers are bombarded with advice from medical experts and laypersons on social media (Johnson & Quinlan, 2019), leaving them feeling pressured to conform to a narrow vision of good motherhood. The ideology of combative mothering (Moore & Abetz, 2016) and circulating discourses such as "breast is best" point to a prevailing notion that there is a single "right way" to mother. Weikle (2023) identified arguments about the "right" way to be a mother on social media pages targeted at mothers, where interactants used various strategies to promote their discourse while silencing others. Such dominant mothering discourses can increase anxiety about personal responsibility, the need to be perfect, a fear of negative evaluation, and a distorted perception of the risks of negative outcomes in parenting (Rowe & Fisher, 2015).

While messages from healthcare providers can be stringent and dehumanized, the reality is that parents don't always follow the prescribed guidelines. There is a lack of guidance from healthcare providers around what to do if your baby won't sleep on their back, or if your baby can't breastfeed, leaving women to feel like failures. Furthermore, prospective parents' intentions to engage in certain parenting practices are connected to their perceived societal norms of those practices; however, those prospective parents do not accurately predict the societal norms of some parenting practices (Powell & Karraker, 2017). For example, Powell and Karraker (2017) found that the majority of prospective parents in their study incorrectly estimated the percentage of mothers who breastfed, the percentage of parents who circumcised their male infants, and the percentage of parents who co-slept with their infants. These inaccurate perceptions may impact mothers' well-being if they perceive they are unable to live up to not only their own intentions, but the societal standards they wish to meet.

However, there are alternate messages from other communities, such as co-sleeping or "fed is best." These messages may be more likely to take into account the emotional, mental, and physical well-being of the mother. For example, McKenna and Volpe (2007) detail how mothers found many benefits to co-sleeping, and felt co-sleeping is a personal decision, and not one that should be dictated by others, including health professionals. Instead of a "one right way" approach, healthcare providers can take a more inclusive approach, offering a range of options and empowering mothers to find a path that works best for their unique circumstances and that considers the health and safety of the infant. Through offering a range of options, providers can not only guide parents on safety and health practices but also could improve the interpersonal relationship between provider and parent.

Along with the interpersonal relationships pediatricians develop with parents of their patients, mothers develop interpersonal relationships with their own healthcare practitioners, including OBGYNs, nurses, and lactation consultants, among others. In this book, I touched on the interpersonal relationship between healthcare practitioners and mothers when discussing mother's health. The mothers who did not feel supported by their providers described a lack of relational caring. Their experiences further illuminate the benefit of relationship-centered care, or care that recognizes the personhood of both parties, acknowledges emotions, and considers patient expectations and knowledge (Duggan & Thompson, 2011) within the context of maternal health.

As part of the relationship-centered care, healthcare providers and other support persons can talk to moms about how having a child will affect their identity. Healthcare providers usually suggest classes for new parents, but these classes focus on delivery, infant care, and breastfeeding. Parenting classes could add or focus on a changing identity element. Along with pregnant mothers, fathers, partners, and adoptive parents could benefit from learning about how one's sense of self and how others treat them change after having or adopting a child. For example, The Gottman Institute offers "Bringing Baby Home" classes for new parents that focus on emotional connection, intimacy, and conflict management for partners after they become parents.

Furthermore, perhaps a focus on identity can help women manage the uncertainty of their changing self as they experience postpartum depression. Voorhees (2022) argued that illness-related uncertainty can be somewhat alleviated by helping individuals recognize how their illness (in that study's case, chronic pain) influences their sense of self. Similarly, by helping women understand how their postpartum depression may be impacting their sense of self and other aspects of identity, uncertainty can be mitigated.

Finally, postpartum depression remains a stigmatized illness. Rates of postpartum depression in the United States are debatable but generally listed as between one in eight and one in five women. Still, the rate of women who experience elevated postpartum depressive symptoms is much higher, at around 60 percent (Beck et al., 2011). When healthcare practitioners talk about postpartum depression as something rare, and when relational partners and healthcare providers dismiss mothers who disclose symptoms, mothers are more likely to think there is something morally and permanently wrong with them rather than understanding that they are experiencing the most common health complication for women following the birth of a child (Rafferty et al., 2019). Hecht (2015) argues that researchers can use a CTI framework to promote positive health behaviors. In the current context, I've used CTI to study this common health complication for mothers—perhaps a focus on identity gaps around postpartum depression can decrease the stigma of the condition, presumably leading to more women seeking treatment.

Through analyzing identity experiences during postpartum depression from a communicative framework, I offer suggestions for healthcare providers on communicating with prenatal and postpartum mothers, based on previous research along with the experiences analyzed for this book. First, take a more empathetic and inclusive approach to discussing child-rearing with parents and focus on relationship-centered care for mothers. Second, consider identity experiences when discussing changes women and parents may face as they become new mothers/parents and when recommending parenting classes. Finally, normalize seeking help for postpartum depression by discussing the mental health conditions mothers face postpartum as common health complications rather than rare occurrences. Next, I discuss how healthcare professionals, educators, and parental experts can incorporate support persons into discussions about postpartum depression education and support.

Practical Application for Parental Education Specialists and Healthcare Education Specialists: Target Support Persons in Postpartum Depression Education and Support

The two persons most discussed in my interviews (with majority heterosexual cisgender women in opposite sex marriages) were male spouses and mothers of the mother. Women mentioned both their spouses and their mother being supportive when they were discussing the challenges they faced. Additionally, mothers discussed tensions they faced within these relationships. Through the lens of CTI, I conceptualized these tensions as relational and communal identity gaps. Considering gaps related to the relational layer of identity is significant, because within CTI, other's perceptions of us, received through communication, are not just an influence on our selves, but actually part of our selves (Jung & Hecht, 2008).

Within the current context, messages from others constitute part of how women thought of themselves as mothers. When women receive unsupportive messages or messages that conflict with self-concept, identity gaps may form. Considering gaps related to the communal layer of identity is significant because the communal identity of mother is not only present in mother's own identity, but as communal identities are societal, is also present in other's conceptualizations of mother and therefore, other's ascribed identities on mothers. This has implications for whom healthcare providers and parental education specialists target for postpartum depression support. Support structures and education tools can be developed not just for mothers, but also for those within their support system. Researchers have identified social support as a key factor in preventing postpartum depression (Vik & DeGroot, 2021), so it makes sense to target support persons.

If relational partners can be taught how to provide support to new mothers, perhaps postpartum depression, or at least the severity of it, can be mitigated. Fathers could also be encouraged to handle the majority of childcare during the six-week recovery period after birth, so mothers can focus on healing and breastfeeding (if they choose to breastfeed). Furthermore, "partners who encourage mothers to seek help when they are experiencing challenges early in the postpartum period may potentially assist in preventing postpartum depression" (Dennis & Chung-Lee, 2006, p. 326). Healthcare campaigns also can focus on helping fathers to learn how to talk to their partner about seeking treatment for postpartum depression. Indeed, fathers may lack knowledge to support their partner in postpartum depression (Henshaw et al., 2016).

Another important source of support for new mothers is their own mother, according to the women I interviewed. As ideas about parenting and maternal mental health are changing, another focus for health campaigns could be on educating mothers/mother figures of the mother on childcare, the struggles mothers face today, and perinatal mood disorders and how to treat them. For example, in their study on mother/daughter dyads and breast cancer, Fisher and Wolf (2019) conclude that health interventions focused on educating family members about gendered ideologies related to women's and mother's responsibilities could influence how family members respond to mothers' health crises. While their study focused on breast cancer, the overall problems faced by women align with the problems mothers faced in the current study—family member's ideologies of womanhood and motherhood influenced how they responded to the postpartum depression symptoms or diagnosis. However, it is important to note that overall, most of the women I spoke with saw their mothers as supportive.

Practical Advice for New Mothers: Reframe the Stigma around Postpartum Depression

Much of research on postpartum depression focuses on the negative outcomes of untreated and undiagnosed postpartum depression for mothers and children. Importantly, the experiences shared in this book show that postpartum depression can have a positive lasting impact. I argue that this is an important contribution to the conversation about postpartum depression and how we approach the topic as researchers in and beyond the field of communication studies. Postpartum depression is a negatively veiled experience, even in research. And while that is understandable, one can speculate that it may lead a mother to panic or experience more anxiety when she is diagnosed with postpartum depression or lead her to not seek care. However, my work here points to positive outcomes of women's experiences on their selves, their relationships, and their communities. Furthermore, the women I spoke with were taking actionable steps to change the stigma and lack of knowledge associated with postpartum depression, which also has a positive impact on maternal mental health overall. I hope these outcomes bring light to the fact that a diagnosis of postpartum depression does not mean you have failed your child or that the world is over.

Colaner et al. (2014) concluded in their study on adoptive identity that it is possible that identity gaps can initiate positive identity change. In the current context, identity gaps may have had immediate negative impacts; however, even negative experiences seemed to at times have lasting positive impacts on women's identities. For example, while a relational-relational gap may have initially brought conflict into a marital relationship, that same relationship was sometimes described as having improved as a result of the shared struggle of postpartum depression. Indeed, over time, identity gaps may no longer be negative as individuals find ways to cope with the gaps (Maeda & Hecht, 2012).

The information shared in this book should be encouraging for mothers in several ways. First, mothers who experience postpartum depression may feel additional anxiety about the effects their postpartum depression will have on their children or their long-term selves. However, the women I spoke with felt a positive lasting impact on themselves and their relationships. Second, mothers are inundated with messages on how they should mother and how to be a mother. By understanding that these messages are socially constructed, mothers can manage those messages that are damaging to their identity and experiences. Third, the experiences related to disclosure should be encouraging to mothers who may be experiencing postpartum depression—all the mothers in the current study who disclosed their postpartum depression received supportive messages from other moms, whether that was their own mom or other mothers. There are ways to find support as one experiences postpartum depression. While women still experience judgment related to their symptoms or diagnosis, ideas about postpartum depression seem to be shifting.

In Summary

In the fall of 2024, the US Surgeon General issued a public health advisory on parental mental health and well-being. In the report, Surgeon General Vivek H. Murthy discusses recent research on parental stress and the parental load, citing a recent study by the American Psychological Association reporting that 48 percent of parents say their stress is "completely overwhelming" most days (APA, 2023, as cited in Murthy, 2024). The report points to shame and guilt as emotions that can negatively impact mental health (Murthy, 2024) and discusses how societal expectations and pressures to meet an ideal parenting standard can contribute to stress, which in turn can have negative impacts on mental health and well-being (Murthy, 2024). The stakes are high. The standards are impossible to meet.

And yet, as mothers, we feel failure when we can't live up to these impossible standards. The standards, expectations, and messages from others infiltrate our identities, and our sense of self falters. We ask ourselves that same question Miranda put in his song: "Who am I if I don't have what it takes?" By understanding identity as communicative and manifesting in more than just a sense of self but in relationships, enacted behaviors, and larger ideologies, we can get a better picture of the impact of postpartum depression on identity. Now more than ever, we need to recognize how mental health

illnesses, including postpartum depression, are impacted by cultural norms, relationships, and messages from others. The advisory calls on researchers to conduct in-depth, qualitative work to better understand parents' experiences. I hope this book advances understanding of women's postpartum experiences a little more, furthering the recognition of the importance of communication and interaction in identity construction, well-being, mental health, and cultural norms.

Chapter Summary

Educators and healthcare providers should extend their parent preparation education beyond the physical care of the infant and into the well-being and mental care of parents. Understanding the change one is about to go through may help women better navigate the complexities of postpartum life. Postpartum depression is not rare. In fact, it is the most common health complication following the birth of one's child. By understanding postpartum depression as a common complication, we can break the stigma and encourage more women to seek support. We need to target support persons in postpartum depression education. Spouses and mothers of the mother were important support persons for the women I interviewed. There is life beyond postpartum depression. While experiencing it, women may lose hope that they will ever feel like themselves again. However, the women I spoke with talked about the positive outcomes on their relationships and themselves along with the hard parts. The US Surgeon General recently released a public health advisory pointing to parental stress, mental health, and well-being as a public health issue. Through understanding how communication impacts our well-being and mental health, we can better take action collectively and individually to address this public health concern.

Afterword

Throughout the book, I shared some of my own experience with postpartum depression. I was diagnosed with postpartum depression by my OBGYN after the birth of my second child. Like some of the other women mentioned in this book, I didn't tell anyone I had postpartum depression. I didn't tell my parents or my friends. I think the first person outside of my husband that I told was a good friend who had kids the same age as me and who I knew had gone through some postpartum depression. Slowly, I let it trickle out. It wasn't so much that I wanted this person to know or this person not to know, it was just that disclosing this experience was face-threatening for me (although I didn't understand that enough to explicate it at the time). I wanted to be perceived as perfect and as a good mom by my friends. I still wanted my parents' approval, even though I was in my early thirties. I finally told my parents after I felt like my normal self again. I was on anxiety medication which was my saving grace. I mentioned it briefly, in a "hey this happened to me, but you don't need to worry because I'm fine now," way, and didn't talk about it much more than that. Now that I've been engaged in this research for years, I make a conscious effort to share my experience more. It is still face-threatening, but I believe that small conversations can make big changes in attitudes, stigma, and prevailing ideologies. I can't quantify how many times I've told a fellow mom friend, or mom acquaintance, about my dissertation topic and learned that they also experienced postpartum depression. Small conversations have impact.

So, how did I recover from postpartum depression? First and foremost, medicine. I was scared to take medicine, but I'm so glad I did. But I think another event helped propel me out of my depression. I got into and started grad school. I was able to make the career move I had been dreaming of for years. I started my PhD program when my son was barely one year old, and my daughter had just turned four. Finding my vocational fulfillment undoubtedly helped me through the postpartum depression. I am a better mom because of my career.

I feel a deep sense of gratitude to those who have come before me to share their stories and talk about PMDs. I can say with 100 percent certainty that the reason I am able to write this reflection, the reason I am able to do the research I am doing, is because some of the stigma surrounding PMDs is gone. There is certainly a lot still there, but conversations are happening and attitudes are changing enough that I can write this without a deep fear that I will be stigmatized (some certainly will judge, but not all). That doesn't mean I don't worry about how others perceive me as a mother. As I wrote this text, I constantly thought in the back of my mind, "I hope that whoever reads doesn't get the idea that I do not like being a mother." Because while this is an interpretive study first and foremost, I do offer critiques of some of the discourses of motherhood. However, an important distinction is that I am critiquing the social discourses and performance of mothering embedded in society, not the actual experience of being a mother.

I was a mother before I was an academic. And while we have known for a while in academia about the stark differences between the performance of motherhood and the lived experience of motherhood, my own experience and the talk of my participants suggest that these ideas are not prevalent in mainstream culture. As I have been able to learn about how motherhood is socially constructed, I've been able to let go of the ideologies that were not serving myself, my children, or my marriage, and that has led to me finding myself in motherhood more than ever, and feeling true joy and confidence in being a mother. Ultimately, I hope this work helps us re-define motherhood, so current and future mothers, with or without postpartum depression, know that they are not alone, they are worthy, and they don't have to fit in to a certain experience in order to be the best mother for their children.

Appendix

A Brief Description of Method

I approached this research from an interpretive paradigm, influenced by the intergroup communication perspective and feminist theories. The research process was conducted in the summer and fall of 2021. After receiving IRB approval from my university, I used a purposeful sampling strategy to recruit women who either had experienced or were experiencing postpartum depression, were over the age of eighteen, and who had a child within the last ten years. Participants did not need a clinical diagnosis of postpartum depression to participate. I recruited participants by working with a regional postpartum support organization, a local mother's group, a local counseling and therapy clinic, and shared my recruitment script on my personal social media accounts (all approved by IRB). After receiving signed consent, I interviewed participants via Zoom (due to Covid-19 research restrictions at the time). I interviewed a total of sixteen women.

Racially, participants identified as white (N=13), Black or African American (N=2), and Southeast Asian (N=1). Participants identified as straight (N=14), Queer and Bisexual (N=1), and Straight and Questioning (N=1), and were married (N=14), single (N=1), and divorced (N=1). All married participants were married to the father of their child(ren). Participants' age ranged between twenty-seven and forty-two years old (M=33.75, SD=4.15). Most participants had one living child (N=9), while other participants had two (N=6) or three (N=1) living children. Participants' children were between seven-week-olds and eleven-year-olds.

Most participants were college educated, either with a bachelor's degree (N=6), master's degree (N=6), some graduate work (N=1), or JD, MD, PhD, or other terminal degree (N=1). One participant's highest level of education was a high school degree, and one participant did not answer. Participants' total household income ranged from $40,000 to $99,999 (N=7), $100,000 to $199,999 (N=5), under $40,000 (N=2), and $200,000 or above (N=1), with one participant not answering. Religiously, participants identified as Christian (N=4), Catholic (N=2), and Islamic (N=1). Six participants identified as not practicing or did not answer the question.

To analyze my data, I used Tracy's (2020) phronetic iterative approach to analysis. This approach accounts for using theory as a sensitizing framework while also leaving room for interpretation beyond the theory or framing the results in a way that can offer practical solutions. I drew on Braun and Clarke (2006) for guidelines on thematic analysis and on Charmaz (2014) and Baxter (2011) for other guidelines on interpretive research. Inherent to interpretive study is a back-and-forth between transcription, coding, writing, data collection, memo writing, and other analytical procedures. I transcribed all interview data myself with the assistance of the Microsoft Word automatic transcription tool, ending with a total of 249 single-spaced transcribed pages. During the transcription process, I removed all names and replaced them with pseudonyms. I transcribed each interview as soon as possible after recording, usually within a few days of the interview.

Per the phronetic iterative analysis approach, I engaged in primary, secondary, and axial coding. I used NVivo software to organize my coding process. Writing a draft of my results was the most helpful in understanding how I had interpreted my data, so as I began my results draft, I collapsed, expanded, and renamed codes. As I moved through each cycle of coding, I wrote memos. Finally, I engaged in member reflections.

To ensure research quality, I based my methodological procedures on Tracy's (2020) eight "big tent" criteria for high-quality qualitative research. I find the "big tent" framework an effective and useful standard to evaluate high-quality qualitative research because of its comprehensiveness in capturing all aspects of the qualitative research process and its focus on both the end goals for quality and the means to achieve the end goals. Tracy's "big tent" criteria are: worthiness of topic, rich rigor, sincerity, credibility, resonance, significant contribution, ethical, and meaningful coherence.

Study Limitations

Despite the contributions of the findings, this study does present limitations, as with all research. The study is limited in scope—I caution scholars and other readers from extending these findings beyond their scope. This study is an interpretive, qualitative study; therefore, while the findings are useful, they are not statistically generalizable. The homogeny of the participants in regard to race, gender, sexual orientation, and family structure, among other traits, limits the diversity of the experiences that could be explored. However, this does not mean that the experiences reconstructed here are unvaluable or unimportant, only that they represent one picture of women's experiences, not the only picture.

Second, the time in which this research was conducted limited the methodology. I conducted this study during the Covid-19 pandemic. Due to safety constraints on in-person research, I conducted my interviews through video conferencing. The mediated format of the interviews may have led to different types of interactions than a face-to-face environment would have, as appearance, body language, and context can affect the interview process (Charmaz, 2014). Second, the Covid-19 pandemic strain on women, and mothers in particular, meant I faced recruitment challenges as I asked participants for an hour of their time, unpaid. I had nine participants cancel or not show up to their interview time, and hearing from them may have provided deeper or varied insight into some of the experiences I explored. The Covid-19 pandemic restrictions also impacted my own life as I struggled to situate my research, teaching, and home life within the limitations and uncertainty of that time.

Finally, recruiting through postpartum support groups meant I was able to find participants who had experienced postpartum depression; however, it also likely means that their postpartum depression was a salient part of their identity and that they sought to support that identity. I later recruited through social media but did not get as many participants from those recruitment efforts. Therefore, other women who did not consider postpartum depression to be salient to their experience or identities may have different experiences and identity manifestations than the ones described in this work. We know that many women who experience postpartum depression do not disclose their postpartum depression and go undiagnosed and untreated, and it stands to reason that their experience may be different than what was reconstructed here. Furthermore, mothers who had a more "favorable" experience with postpartum depression may have selected the study over other who had a harder time (although many of the mothers in the study struggled significantly with their postpartum depression).

References

Abdollahi, F., Lye, M.-S., Md Zain, A., Shariff Ghazali, S., & Zarghami, M. (2011). Postnatal depression and its associated factors in women from different cultures. *Iranian Journal of Psychiatry and Behavioral Sciences*, 5(2), 5–11.

Abrams, L. S., & Curran, L. (2011). Maternal identity negotiations among low-income women with symptoms of postpartum depression. *Qualitative Health Research*, 21(3), 373–85. https://doi.org/10.1177/1049732310385123.

Afifi, T. D., & Harrison, K. (2018). Theory of resilience and relational load (TRRL): Understanding families as systems of stress and calibration. In D. O. Braithwaite, E. A. Suter, & K. Floyd (Eds.), *Engaging theories in family communication* (2nd ed., pp. 324–36). Routledge.

Alford, A. M. (2019). Mothering and motherhood: Socially constructing the role of mothers. In A. M. Alford & M. Miller-Day (Eds.), *Constructing motherhood and daughterhood across the lifespan* (pp. 37–56). Peter Lang.

American Psychological Association (APA) (2023, November). *Infographic: Stress of parents compared to other adults*. https://www.apa.org/news/press/releases/stress/2023/infographics/infographicparents-other-adults.

Aswad, J. (2022, December 3). Lin-Manuel Miranda on the surprise success of "We Don't Talk About Bruno". *Variety*. Accessed June 25, 2024. https://variety.com/2022/music/news/lin-manuel-miranda-we-dont-talk-about-bruno-encanto-1235448749/.

Athan, A. M. (2024). A critical need for the concept of matrescence in perinatal psychiatry. *Frontiers in Psychiatry*, 15, 1–7. https://doi.org/10.3389/fpsyt.2024.1364845.

Bailey, Z. D., Krieger, N., Agénor, M., Graves, J., Linos, N., & Bassett, M. T. (2017). Structural racism and health inequities in the USA: Evidence and interventions. *The Lancet*, 389(10077), 1453–63. https://doi.org/10.1016/S0140-6736(17)30569-X.

Bauman, B. L., Ko, J. Y., Cox, S., D'Angelo, D. V., Warner, L., Folger, S., Tevendale, H. D., Coy, K. C., Harrison, L., & Barfield, W. D. (2020). Vital signs: Postpartum depressive symptoms and provider discussions about perinatal depression—United States, 2018. *MMWR. Morbidity and Mortality Weekly Report*, 69(19), 575–81. https://doi.org/10.15585/mmwr.mm6919a2.

Baxter, L. A. (2011). *Voicing relationships: A dialogic perspective*. Sage.
Beck, C. T. (1993). Teetering on the edge: A substantive theory of postpartum depression. *Nursing Research*, 42(1), 42–8.
Beck, C. T. (2002). Postpartum depression: A metasynthesis. *Qualitative Health Research*, 12(4), 453–72. https://doi.org/10.3928/0048-5713-20050701-04.
Beck, C. T. (2006). Postpartum depression: It isn't just the blues. *The American Journal of Nursing*, 106(5), 40–51.
Beck, C. T., Records, K., & Rice, M. (2006). Further development of the postpartum depression predictors inventory-revised. *Journal of Obstetric, Gynecologic, and Neonatal Nursing*, 35(6), 735–45. https://doi.org/10.1111/J.1552-6909.2006.00094.x.
Beck, C. T., Gable, R. K., Sakala, C., & Declercq, E. R. (2011). Postpartum depressive symptomatology: Results from a two-stage U.S. national survey. *Journal of Midwifery and Women's Health*, 56(5), 427–35. https://doi.org/10.1111/j.1542-2011.2011.00090.x.
Bergquist, G., Soliz, J., Everhart, K., Braithwaite, D. O., & Kreimer, L. (2019). Investigating layers of identity and identity gaps in refugee resettlement experiences in the midwestern United States. *Western Journal of Communication*, 83(3), 383–402. https://doi.org/10.1080/10570314.2018.1552009.
Braun, V., & Clarke, V. (2006). Using thematic analysis in psychology. *Qualitative Research in Psychology*, 3(2), 77–101. https://doi.org/10.1191/1478088706qp0 63oa.
Canty, L. (2022). The lived experience of severe maternal morbidity among Black women. *Nursing Inquiry*, 29(1), 1–15. https://doi.org/10.1111/nin.12466.
Centers for Disease Control (2021). *Depression among women*. Retrieved March 25, 2021, from https://www.cdc.gov/reproductivehealth/depression/index.htm.
Charmaz, K. (2014). *Constructing grounded theory* (2nd ed.). Sage.
Choi, S. Y., Venetis, M. K., Greene, K., Magsamen-Conrad, K., Checton, M. G., & Banerjee, S. C. (2016). Planning a stigmatized nonvisible illness disclosure: Applying the disclosure decision-making model. *Journal of Psychology: Interdisciplinary and Applied*, 150(8), 1004–25. https://doi.org/10.1080/00223980.2016.1226742.
Colaner, C. W., Halliwell, D., & Guignon, P. (2014). "What do you say to your mother when your mother's standing beside you?" Birth and adoptive family contributions to adoptive identity via relational identity and relational–relational identity gaps. *Communication Monographs*, 81(4), 469–94. https://doi.org/10.1080/03637751.2014.955808.

Constantinou, G., Varela, S., & Buckby, B. (2021). Reviewing the experiences of maternal guilt – the "Motherhood Myth" influence. *Health Care for Women International*, 42(4–6), 852–76. https://doi.org/10.1080/07399332.2020.1835917.

Craig, R. T. (2018). For a practical discipline. *Journal of Communication*, 68(2), 289–97. https://doi.org/10.1093/joc/jqx013.

Cronin-Fisher, V., & Parcell, E. S. (2019). Making sense of dissatisfaction during the transition to motherhood through relational dialectics theory. *Journal of Family Communication*, 19(2), 157–70. https://doi.org/10.1080/15267431.2019.1590364.

DeGroot, J. M., & Vik, T. A. (2019). "Fake smile. Everything is under control": The flawless performance of motherhood. *Western Journal of Communication*, 85(1), 42–60. https://doi.org/10.1080/10570314.2019.1678763.

DeGroot, J. M., & Vik, T. A. (2020). "The weight of our household rests on my shoulders": Inequity in family work. *Journal of Family Issues*, 41(8), 1258–81. https://doi.org/10.1177/0192513X19887767.

Dennis, C. L., & Chung-Lee, L. (2006). Postpartum depression help-seeking barriers and maternal treatment preferences: A qualitative systematic review. *Birth*, 33(4), 323–31. https://doi.org/10.1111/J.1523-536X.2006.00130.X.

Duggan, A. P., & Thompson, T. L. (2011). Provider-patient interaction and related outcomes. In T. L. Thomspon, R. Parrott, & J. F. Nussbaum (Eds.), *The Routledge handbook of health communication* (pp. 414–27). Routledge.

Eddy, B., Poll, V., Whiting, J., & Clevesy, M. (2019). Forgotten fathers: Postpartum depression in men. *Journal of Family Issues*, 40(8), 1001–17. https://doi.org/10.1177/0192513X19833111.

Elliott, G. K., Millard, C., & Sabroe, I. (2020). The utilization of cultural movements to overcome stigma in narrative of postnatal depression. *Frontiers in Psychiatry*, 11(October), 1–13. https://doi.org/10.3389/fpsyt.2020.532600.

Faulkner, S. L., & Hecht, M. L. (2011). The negotiation of closetable identities: A narrative analysis of lesbian, gay, bisexual, transgendered queer Jewish identity. *Journal of Social and Personal Relationships*, 28(6), 829–47. https://doi.org/10.1177/0265407510391338.

Fenwick, J., Barclay, L., & Schmied, V. (2008). Craving closeness: A grounded theory analysis of women's experiences of mothering in the Special Care Nursery. *Women and Birth*, 21(2), 71–85. https://doi.org/10.1016/J.WOMBI.2008.03.006.

Fisher, C. L., & Wolf, B. M. (2019). Understanding mother-daughter communication and health through a discourse of "responsible womanhood." In A. M. Alford & M. Miller-Day (Eds.), *Constructing motherhood and daughterhood across the lifespan* (pp. 265–80). Peter Lang.

Glenn, E. N. (1994). Social constructions of mothering: A thematic overview. In E. N. Glenn, G. Chang, & L. R. Forcey (Eds.), *Mothering: Ideology, experience, agency* (pp. 1–32). Routledge.

Goffman, E. (1959). *The presentation of self in everyday life*. Anchor Books.

Greenaway, K. H., Gallois, C., & Haslam, S. A. (2018). Social psychological approaches to intergroup communication. In H. Giles & J. Harwood (Eds.), *The Oxford encyclopedia of intergroup communication* (pp. 367–79). Oxford University Press.

Hadfield, H., & Wittkowski, A. (2017). Women's experiences of seeking and receiving psychological and psychosocial interventions for postpartum depression: A systematic review and thematic synthesis of the qualitative literature. *Journal of Midwifery & Women's Health*, 62, 723–36. https://doi.org/10.1111/jmwh.12669.

Hays, S. (1996). *The cultural contradictions of motherhood*. Yale University Press.

Hecht, M. L. (1993). 2002 - A research odyssey: Toward the development of a communication theory of identity. *Communication Monographs*, 60, 76–82. https://doi.org/10.1080/03637759309376297.

Hecht, M. L. (2015). Communication theory of identity: Multilayered understandings of performed identities. In D. O. Braithwaite & P. Schrodt (Eds.), *Engaging theories in interpersonal communication: Multiple perspectives* (2nd ed., pp. 175–87). Sage.

Hecht, M. L., Warren, J. R., Jung, E., & Krieger, J. L. (2005). The communication theory of identity: Development, theoretical perspective, and future directions. In W. B. Gudykunst (Ed.), *Theorizing about intercultural communication* (pp. 257–78). Sage.

Henshaw, E. J., Durkin, K. M., & Snell, R. J. (2016). First-time parents' shared representation of postpartum depressive symptoms: A qualitative analysis. *Social Science and Medicine*, 160, 102–10. https://doi.org/10.1016/j.socscimed.2016.05.025.

Hessami, K., Romanelli, C., Chiurazzi, M., & Cozzolino, M. (2020). COVID-19 pandemic and maternal mental health: A systematic review and meta-analysis. *Journal of Maternal-Fetal and Neonatal Medicine*, 35(20), 4014–21. https://doi.org/10.1080/14767058.2020.1843155.

Holman, L., & McKeever, R. (2017). The Andrea Yates effect: Priming mental illness stereotypes through exemplification of postpartum disorders. *Health Communication*, 32(10), 1284–96. https://doi.org/10.1080/10410236.2016.1219929.

Hosek, A. M., Mattys, H., & Weikle, K. M. (2021). From "breast is best" to "your choice": Memorable messages mothers receive about breastfeeding. In A. Cooke-

Jackson & V. Rubinsky (Eds.), *Communicating intimate health* (pp. 171–86). Lexington Books.

Johnson, B. L., & Quinlan, M. M. (2019). *You're doing it wrong! Mothering, media, and medical expertise*. Rutgers University Press.

Jung, E. (2011). Identity gap: Mediator between communication input and outcome variables. *Communication Quarterly*, 59(3), 315–38. https://doi.org/10.1080/01463373.2011.583501.

Jung, E., & Hecht, M. L. (2004). Elaborating the communication theory of identity: Identity gaps and communication outcomes. *Communication Quarterly*, 52(3), 265–83. https://doi.org/10.1080/01463370409370197.

Jung, E., & Hecht, M. L. (2008). Identity gaps and level of depression among Korean immigrants. *Health Communication*, 23(4), 313–25. https://doi.org/10.1080/10410230802229688.

Jung, E., Hecht, M. L., & Wadsworth, B. C. (2007). The role of identity in international students' psychological well-being in the United States: A model of depression level, identity gaps, discrimination, and acculturation. *International Journal of Intercultural Relations*, 31(5), 605–24. https://doi.org/10.1016/j.ijintrel.2007.04.001.

Kam, J. A., & Hecht, M. L. (2009). Investigating the role of identity gaps among communicative and relational outcomes within the grandparent-grandchild relationship: The young-adult grandchildren's perspective. *Western Journal of Communication*, 73(4), 456–80. https://doi.org/10.1080/10570310903279067.

Kennedy-Lightsey, C. D., Martin, M. M., LaBelle, S., & Weber, K. (2015). Attachment, identity gaps, and communication and relational outcomes in marital couples' public performances. *Journal of Family Communication*, 15(3), 232–48. https://doi.org/10.1080/15267431.2015.1043430.

Knapp, M. L., Stohl, C., & Reardon, K. K. (1981). "Memorable" messages. *Journal of Communication*, 31(4), 27–41. https://doi.org/10.1111/j.1460-2466.1981.tb00448.x.

Kozhimannil, K. B., Trinacty, C. M., Busch, A. B., Huskamp, H. A., & Adams, A. S. (2011). Racial and ethnic disparities in postpartum depression care among low-income women. *Psychiatric Services (Washington, D.C.)*, 62(6), 619. https://doi.org/10.1176/APPI.PS.62.6.619.

Maeda, E., & Hecht, M. L. (2012). Identity search: Interpersonal relationships and relational identities of always-single Japanese women over time. *Western Journal of Communication*, 76(1), 44–64. https://doi.org/10.1080/10570314.2012.637539.

McBride, M. C. (2018). Facework theory: Performing familial roles in everyday interactions. In D. O. Braithwaite, E. A. Suter, & K. Floyd (Eds.), *Engaging theories in family communication* (2nd ed., pp. 132–41). Routledge.

McHenry, K. A., & Schultz, D. L. (2014). Skinny jeans: Perfection and competition in motherhood. In L. R. Ennis (Ed.), *Intensive mothering: The cultural contradictions of modern motherhood* (pp. 169–76). Demeter Press.

McKenna, J. J., & Volpe, L. E. (2007). Sleeping with baby: An internet-based sampling of parental experiences, choices, perceptions, and interpretations in a western industrialized context. *Infant and Child Development*, 16(4), 359–85. https://doi.org/10.1002/ICD.525.

McMahon, C., Trapolini, T., & Barnett, B. (2008). Maternal state of mind regarding attachment predicts persistence of postnatal depression in the preschool years. *Journal of Affective Disorders*, 107(1–3), 199–203. https://doi.org/10.1016/j.jad.2007.07.017.

Miranda, L.M., Franco, G., & Encanto Cast (2021). Surface pressure [Song]. On *Encanto* (Original motion picture soundtrack). Walt Disney Records; Disney Enterprises.

Mollard, E. K. (2014). A qualitative meta-synthesis and theory of postpartum depression. *Issues in Mental Health Nursing*, 35(9), 656–63. https://doi.org/10.3109/01612840.2014.893044.

Moore, J., & Abetz, J. (2016). "Uh oh. Cue the [new] mommy wars": The ideology of combative mothering in popular U.S. newspaper articles about attachment parenting. *Southern Communication Journal*, 81(1), 49–62. https://doi.org/10.1080/1041794X.2015.1076026.

Murthy, V. H. (2024). *Parents under pressure: The U.S. Surgeon General's advisory on the mental health & well-being of parents*. U.S. Department of Health and Human Services. https://www.hhs.gov/sites/default/files/parents-under-pressure.pdf.

National Institute of Mental Health (2024). *Postpartum depression facts*. Accessed August 26, 2024. https://www.nimh.nih.gov/health/publications/perinatal-depression/index.shtml.

Nidey, N., Tabb, K. M., Carter, K. D., Bao, W., Strathearn, L., Rohlman, D. S., Wehby, G., & Ryckman, K. (2020). Rurality and risk of perinatal depression among women in the United States. *Journal of Rural Health*, 36(1), 9–16. https://doi.org/10.1111/jrh.12401.

Pagan, C. N. (2018). When doctors downplay women's health concerns. *New York Times*. https://www.nytimes.com/2018/05/03/well/live/when-doctors-downplay-womens-health-concerns.html.

Palladino, E., Varin, M., Lary, T., & Baker, M. M. (2020). Thoughts of self-harm and associated risk factors among postpartum women in Canada. *Journal of Affective Disorders*, 270, 69–74. https://doi.org/10.1016/j.jad.2020.03.054.

Palmer-Wackerly, A. L., Dailey, P. M., Krok-Schoen, J. L., Rhodes, N. D., & Krieger, J. L. (2018). Patient perceptions of illness identity in cancer clinical trial decision-making. *Health Communication*, 33(8), 1045–54. https://doi.org/10.1080/10410236.2017.1331189.

Postpartum Support International (PSI) (2024). *Perinatal mental health*. https://www.postpartum.net/perinatal-mental-health/.

Powell, D. N., & Karraker, K. (2017). Prospective parents' knowledge about parenting and their anticipated child-rearing decisions. *Family Relations*, 66(3), 453–67. https://doi.org/10.1111/FARE.12259.

Rafferty, J., Mattson, G., Earls, M. F., & Yogman, M. W. (2019). Incorporating recognition and management of perinatal depression into pediatric practice. *Pediatrics*, 143(1), 31. https://doi.org/e20183260.

Rittenour, C. E., & Odenweller, K. G. (2019). It's not that easy: Challenges of motherhood. In A. M. Alford & M. Miller-Day (Eds.), *Constructing motherhood and daughterhood across the lifespan* (pp. 251–64). Peter Lang.

Rowe, H. J., & Fisher, J. R. W. (2015). Do contemporary social and health discourses arouse peripartum anxiety? A qualitative investigation of women's accounts. *Women's Studies International Forum*, 51, 56–65. https://doi.org/10.1016/j.wsif.2015.05.002.

Rubinsky, V., & Cooke-Jackson, A. (2017). "Tell me something other than to use a condom and sex is scary": Memorable messages women and gender minorities wish for and recall about sexual health. *Women's Studies in Communication*, 40(4), 379–400. https://doi.org/10.1080/07491409.2017.1368761.

Scharp, K. M., & Thomas, L. J. (2017). "What would a loving mom do today?": Exploring the meaning of motherhood in stories of prenatal and postpartum depression. *Journal of Family Communication*, 17(4), 401–14. https://doi.org/10.1080/15267431.2017.1355803.

Seymour-Smith, M., Cruwys, T., Haslam, S. A., & Brodribb, W. (2017). Loss of group memberships predicts depression in postpartum mothers. *Social Psychiatry and Psychiatric Epidemiology*, 52(2), 201–10. https://doi.org/10.1007/s00127-016-1315-3.

Slomian, J., Honvo, G., Emonts, P., Reginster, J. Y., & Bruyère, O. (2019). Consequences of maternal postpartum depression: A systematic review of maternal and infant outcomes. *Women's Health*, 15, 1–55. https://doi.org/10.1177/1745506519844044.

Soliz, J., & Colaner, C. W. (2018). Communication accommodation theory and communication theory of identity. In D. O. Braithwaite, E. A. Suter, & K. Floyd (Eds.), *Engaging theories in family communication* (2nd ed., pp. 75–86). Routledge.

Swain, J. E., Kim, P., & Ho, S. S. (2011). Neuroendocrinology of parental response to baby-cry. *Journal of Neuroendocrinology*, 23(11), 1036–41. https://doi.org/10.1111/J.1365-2826.2011.02212.X.

Tajfel, H. (1974). Social identity and intergroup behavior. *Social Science Inform*, 13(2), 65–93.

Tosun, L. P., Öztürk, A., & Özdemir, G. (2020). Mother to mother: Mothers' social comparison-based emotions on social networking sites. *Europe's Journal of Psychology*, 16(4), 602–18. https://doi.org/10.5964/ejop.v16i4.2159.

Tracy, S. J. (2020). *Qualitative research methods* (2nd ed.). Wiley Blackwell.

Vik, K., & Hafting, M. (2012). "Smile through it!" Keeping up the facade while suffering from postnatal depressive symptoms and feelings of loss: Findings of a qualitative study. *Psychology*, 3(9), 810–17. https://doi.org/10.4236/psych.2012.329123.

Vik, T. A., & DeGroot, J. M. (2021). "I don't let everyone see my struggles": Mothers' social support and privacy management. *Personal Relationships*, 28(3), 475–94. https://doi.org/10.1111/pere.12372.

Voorhees, H. L. (2022). "I was literally just not myself": How chronic pain changes multiple frames of identity. *Health Communication*, 38(8), 1641–53. https://doi.org/10.1080/10410236.2022.2025702.

Wagner, P. E., Kunkel, A., & Compton, B. L. (2016). (Trans)lating identity: Exploring discursive strategies for navigating the tensions of identity gaps. *Communication Quarterly*, 64(3), 251–72. https://doi.org/10.1080/01463373.2015.1103286.

Weikle, K. M. (2023). "Have you been in this position? Because your comment does not make sense." Discourse strategies and situated ideals of interaction on social networking sites for mothers. *Western Journal of Communication*, 87(2), 326–45. https://doi.org/10.1080/10570314.2022.2109723.

Willer, E. K., Krebs, E., Castaneda, N., Hoyt, K. D., Droser, V. A., Johnson, J. A., & Hunniecutt, J. (2020). Our babies['] count[er story]: A narrative ethnography of a baby loss remembrance walk ritual. *Communication Monographs*, 87(2), 179–99. https://doi.org/10.1080/03637751.2019.1666289.

Index

www.ingramcontent.com/pod-product-compliance
Ingram Content Group UK Ltd.
Pitfield, Milton Keynes, MK11 3LW, UK
UKHW020207290926
15470UKWH00001B/55

9 781666 961126